MW01129565

Mind Mapping for Men with Adult ADHD

Daily Brain Exercises and Strategies for a Positive
Transformation to Control Anxious Thoughts,
Improve Concentration, and Productivity

by

Jimmy Taylor

A SELFTRANSFORMATIONPATH BOOK

Table of Contents

As a special offer, I am providing you with an added bonus

To thank you for your purchase, you can download my Empowering Checklist for a Positive Mindset for FREE

To get your copy, please go to: **selftransformationpath.com/free-gift**

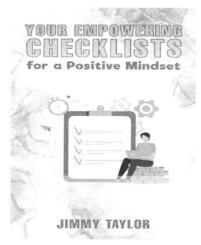

This checklist is designed to provide you with a comprehensive guide to living a happy life in the following areas:

1. Personal Growth and Well-Being

2. Social Connections and Relationships

3. Physical Health and Wellness

4. Leisure and Enjoyment

5. Self-Care and Emotional Well-Being

6. Balanced living

If you want to create a solid foundation for a happy and fulfilling life, make sure to grab a copy of the checklist.

You can also scan this QR code to get access.

Introduction

What lies between where you are and where you want to be sometimes requires traveling through the Twilight Zone.
– Shannon L. Alder

I grew up believing that attention deficit hyperactivity disorder (ADHD) was a condition that affected children. I thought that people grew out of it as they learned emotional regulation, were medicated, or simply developed a tolerance to their symptoms.

What I didn't know was that ADHD is lifelong, and many of us have been living with it without ever realizing something was going on. For adult men, an ADHD diagnosis can be confusing. We've been told that having ADHD means not being able to concentrate, being hyperactive, and having problems controlling our impulses. What we're not told is that ADHD is a spectrum condition that affects people of all ages, and the symptoms of living with ADHD can vary.

For men, ADHD can present as bouts of emotional dysregulation, self-criticism, avoidant behavior, perfectionism, and depression. Our confidence takes a knock as we take on new projects only to never fully complete them. We then berate ourselves, or worse, we hurt the people we love the most.

In fact, the majority of men with ADHD did grow up with the common symptoms associated with the condition, but society deems these behaviors acceptable. Messy or disorganized bedrooms, the inability

1

to sit still and complete tasks, or even keeping a closet tidy are all seen as typical "boy things."

Growing up like this inadvertently reinforces and rewards the behaviors associated with ADHD and ultimately compounds our disappointment in ourselves. We live for the magical moment when we will grow out of the behaviors that get us into trouble, and it's a moment that doesn't come if we never receive a diagnosis and treatment plan.

This justifies the progression of our symptoms and behaviors until we grow up and build different relationships in which our actions, words, and mannerisms cause conflict. We begin to compensate for our difficulties and become defensive of our actions, blaming other people for nagging.

We stigmatize ourselves and become emotionally reactive, all the while intuitively knowing that something is amiss and that there has to be more to life than the whirling thoughts preoccupying our minds.

A diagnosis of ADHD can be both a source of relief and an excuse for our behavior. We can sometimes believe that we are destined to repeat the same cycle because we are broken. The reality is that you *can* thrive! You can take back your life, and you can start today.

I wrote *Mind Mapping for Men with Adult ADHD* as part of my own journey after being diagnosed with ADHD. I, too, had to learn how to stop overthinking, take accountability for my behaviors, and master my ADHD as a superpower I could use to better my career, friendships, and relationships.

Introduction

When reading this book, you can expect to learn how to:

- Gain a deeper understanding of ADHD and how having it uniquely affects you as a man.

- Identify your thought spirals and how to uncover what is fueling your thoughts.

- Mind map for communication clarity and a deeper understanding of your thoughts.

- Plan and successfully take action so that you can achieve your goals.

- Improve your emotional quotient for a better relationship with yourself and others.

Finally, before you continue reading the chapters of this book, I'd like you to know that you're not alone. Men are three times more likely to be diagnosed with ADHD, although not many will seek treatment due to the stigma surrounding it. Approximately 13% of men around the globe will be on the ADHD spectrum, and only 5.4% of men will access formal treatment for their diagnosis.

Having ADHD is nothing to be ashamed of, and it doesn't have to be something that debilitates you for the remainder of your life. You have the power to positively transform your life, calm your anxious thoughts, and improve your concentration and productivity.

Part 1

The ADHD Brain and Overthinking

Chapter 1

Understanding ADHD

What I need is a task. Something to concentrate on, something that will distract me from all the whirling thoughts crowding my head.
– Sylvia Mercedes

Modern medicine may have become far better at diagnosing conditions, disorders, and illnesses, but most of the time, it fails to identify how these syndromes affect men and women differently.

After receiving a diagnosis, we can sometimes feel lost. A prescription in our hand and advice to see a therapist are the only guidance we are given. For some of us, instead of relief, our diagnosis can lead our thoughts to spiral and compound themselves as we ruminate about all the things we think are *wrong* with us.

For others, an ADHD diagnosis comes as a get-out-of-jail-free card for their behaviors and emotional regulation issues. These behaviors can worsen as the newly-diagnosed person feels their actions have a justifiable cause and should be free of criticism. Don't get me wrong; you have no control over your ADHD diagnosis, nor do you have control over having ADHD. However, it does not define you, and you are not a helpless victim trapped in your life and your thoughts.

As you read through this chapter, I'd like you to understand that I am not stereotyping or downplaying the struggles men with ADHD face. ADHD is complex; it falls on a spectrum, which means some of the things you read may apply to you, and others may not.

Unfortunately, ADHD is stigmatized, especially in adults and men. Society places pressure on us to have everything together and be providers for our loved ones. Certain emotions are not welcomed, so often, when we receive a diagnosis, it can become deeply rooted in shame. Defensive behaviors, emotional dysregulation, and angry outbursts can become the center of our existence, which only serves to fuel our deep feelings of inner discomfort.

ADHD in the Neurodiversity Umbrella

Neurodiversity is a word that has gained traction on social media lately, but the concept of being neurodivergent is still not properly understood. We tend to think that being neurodivergent is directly related to autism, which, in itself, is a spectrum disorder.

In reality, neurodiversity is an umbrella term used to define the common neurological characteristics of people with ADHD, autism spectrum disorder, dyslexia, dyspraxia, and dyscalculia.

The point of placing certain disorders under an umbrella term is to help remove stigma and discrimination against people who have them. However, the issue is that when we begin to define people by their condition, we're also defining them by their limitations and deficits.

Having said that, the term neurodiversity does help us to move away from labeling ADHD as a condition associated with weaknesses. It places emphasis on a person's strengths, regardless of whether or not they present with a disorder.

When it comes down to it, everyone has strengths plus weaknesses that limit them, but those who are neurodivergent tend to focus on their limitations because of what they were told when they were younger.

To embrace your ADHD and being neurodivergent, you actively need to work toward shifting your mindset. Move away from the terms "special needs" or "disorder" and toward what you can achieve with the right tools.

Regardless of whether or not you have chosen to be medicated, it's important to move away from operating out of a labeled box filled with guilt and shame.

Without first shifting your mindset and deciding that you're going to tackle ADHD head-on in a strength-based approach, you will never fully understand how focusing on your weaknesses prevents you from using your neurodivergent powers.

Neurodiversity and ADHD in Adults

Being an adult can sometimes feel like a circus juggling act, and the average adult either needs or feels obliged to keep many responsibilities going in order to be functional and successful in their lives.

From parenting to socializing, looking after our mental and physical health, and thriving in our careers, being an adult can be overwhelming, even at the best of times. For those of us with ADHD, this overwhelm can be magnified when we find ourselves constantly late, forgetful, living in disorganized chaos, or generally feeling that everything we have to get done is simply too much.

Avoidance becomes a way of life, and our frustrations manifest through dysregulated emotions, angry outbursts, and waves of anxiety and depression. Science and medicine are not convinced about the exact causes of ADHD. However, the general consensus is that it's a combination of factors, including the environment, the way our brains are hardwired, and a genetic component.

For those of us diagnosed with ADHD at a young age, some of the symptoms we experienced when we were younger will still be prevalent. We may also not be consciously aware of them, as learned behaviors and dysregulation can cause us to become blissfully unaware of our symptoms.

For others, ADHD that is carried into adulthood from childhood can continue to be debilitating. If ADHD was never diagnosed in childhood, our symptoms could feel like a curse that sets us apart from everyone else.

When ADHD is not recognized in childhood, our behaviors are often associated with negative connotations, with adults calling us unruly, defiant, lazy, or just plain bad. This reaffirms in our minds that there is something very wrong with us, and we enter into a deep state of guilt, shame, or even denial.

As a result of denial and the internal stigmas we attach to our ADHD symptoms, we can begin to run into a lot of trouble as adults, and as our responsibilities increase, we drop more and more of the juggling balls. However, it's not that we don't *know* that we need to be organized, focused, regulated, and calm; it's just that the *how* escapes us, further compounding all the negative things we think about ourselves.

The good news is that there is only one difference between adults with ADHD who are thriving and those who are not. They have learned to turn their weaknesses into strengths by accessing the right support, education, and tools.

I want you to know that it's never too late to use your ADHD to your advantage. You can learn how to succeed in life, achieve your goals, and become productive on your own terms.

Your journey to success starts with understanding your symptoms and how they may differ from what you experienced in childhood. Knowing you're not alone and gaining a deeper insight into how ADHD uniquely affects adults will help you better manage your symptoms and begin equipping you with the tools you need.

Types of ADHD

In the past, medicine and psychology recognized three types of ADHD.

These types are:

1. **Combined ADHD**: Characterized by impulsivity and hyperactivity as well as the inability to concentrate. This is the most common form of ADHD.

2. **Impulsive, hyperactive ADHD**: Characterized by impulsive and hyperactive behaviors only, without the inability to concentrate. This is the least common form of ADHD.

3. **Inattentive, distractible ADHD**: Characterized by the inability to pay attention or a high level of distractibility. This form of ADHD is more common in females.

While these three types of ADHD are the most commonly diagnosed and treated, pioneers in behavior and brain disorders have further identified other types of ADHD that can be targeted to help manage the symptoms of ADHD better.

American psychiatrist and brain disorder specialist Dr. Daniel Amen has dedicated his life's work to helping children when diagnosed with ADHD, supporting them to remove the obstacles, and giving them the tools to be successful.

One study conducted by Dr. Amen showed that each of the three types of ADHD could be further broken down into subtypes, each with its own symptoms that required special tools and treatments (Amen, 2001).

It's essential to note that Dr. Amen does not base his research purely on verbal assessments, nor does he rely solely on diagnostic tools. Instead, he uses cutting-edge brain imaging to help identify which areas of the brain are not functioning within a set of normal parameters. By identifying these areas, Dr. Amen can suggest targeted exercises and tools to help the brain work the way it should.

In addition, he discovered that ADHD may affect not only two but three of the brain's neurotransmitters. These neurotransmitters are dopamine, γ-Aminobutyric acid (GABA), and serotonin. Through imaging of the brain, he was also able to find discrepancies in various areas of the brain, not just the prefrontal cortex. In fact, these brain images showed that most of the brain was affected, including the deep structures that help create dopamine.

While Dr. Amen's theories are somewhat controversial and not recognized by medicine just yet, it's important that they are discussed so that you can use the information if you want to (Champ et al., 2021).

Following are the ADHD subtypes that Dr. Amen identified:

- **Classic ADHD** is characterized by distractibility, hyperactivity, inattentiveness, impulsivity, and disorganization.

  Imaging and tests show that this type of ADHD is caused by a dopamine deficiency and not enough blood flow to the cerebellum, basal ganglia, and prefrontal cortex.

- **Inattentive ADHD** is characterized by a shortened attention span, procrastination, perfectionism, daydreaming, introversion, distractibility, and introversion.

  Imaging and testing show that Inattentive ADHD is a symptom of dopamine deficiency as well as having a prefrontal cortex that is not as active as it should be.

- **Overfocused ADHD** presents with the symptoms of classic ADHD but comes with an inability to shift attention or move from task to task easily. People with overfocused ADHD can sometimes become stuck in their thought patterns and behaviors.

Imaging and testing show that this type of ADHD is a result of dopamine and serotonin deficiencies as well as an overactive cingulate gyrus in the brain.

- **Temporal Lobe ADHD** displays all of the symptoms of classic ADHD but also affects memory retention and learning. This ADHD subtype is marked by emotional outbursts, behavioral issues, and risk-taking.

Imaging shows decreased prefrontal cortex activity in those with Temporal Lobe ADHD and some abnormalities in the temporal lobe of the brain.

- **Limbic ADHD** has all of the symptoms of classic ADHD plus a chronic low mood that cannot be characterized as depression. People with Limbic ADHD may also suffer from low energy levels, low self-esteem, and have a "victim mentality."

Imaging shows increased activity in the limbic center of the brain, which affects mood, as well as a decrease in activity in the prefrontal cortex.

- **Ring of Fire ADHD** is characterized by a marked sensitivity to noise, light, and touch. People with this subtype of ADHD may lash out, behave unpredictably, or be anxious and fearful.

Imaging shows a ring of too much activity around the brain's centers, plus increased activity in the cerebral cortex and other areas at times.

- **Anxious ADHD** presents with all of the symptoms of classic ADHD but includes anxious, stressed-out behavior and the physical symptoms of stress.

  Imaging shows that those with Anxious ADHD have an overactive basal ganglia, which can be confusing as other types of ADHD present with low activity in this region of the brain.

Understanding the different types of ADHD and exploring possible subtypes is important because certain medications can actually aggravate the symptoms of specific subtypes. For example, stimulant medications may increase the symptoms associated with Ring of Fire ADHD or Temporal Lobe ADHD.

How Prevalent Is ADHD in Adults

The National Institute of Mental Health study conducted in 2014 showed an overall prevalence of ADHD in adults of around 4.4%.

This percentage was taken as the median between men at 5.4% and women at 3.2%. In adults in the United States (USA), 8.1% of adults between the ages of 18 and 44 had been diagnosed with ADHD (National Institute of Mental Health, 2014).

New studies, however, show a worldwide statistic of 2.8% and only a 0.96% diagnosis in the USA, which is a big difference between the previous 4.4% and 8.1% statistics reported (Song et al., 2021).

There is some debate as to whether or not these statistics are correct, though. Those who agree with them say modern early intervention in children has significantly lowered the number of ADHD cases.

Some schools of thought are more skeptical, saying fewer people are seeking an ADHD diagnosis due to the stigma surrounding it and the bias against people with ADHD.

Diagnosis and Symptoms of ADHD in Adults Versus Kids

Adults with children who have ADHD, as well as adults who suspect they themselves have ADHD, may begin their journey to a formal diagnosis through their general practitioner (GP). While a GP cannot actually give a diagnosis, they can refer you to a specialist for assessment and further investigation into the symptoms you're experiencing. A referral usually occurs after the GP has asked some questions.

These questions will cover:

- What symptoms you are currently experiencing.

- How long you have been experiencing your symptoms.

- The frequency of your symptoms and if they become worse or better while doing certain tasks.

- How your symptoms affect your day-to-day life.

- Whether or not you're experiencing more stress than usual.

- If you have been experiencing other symptoms that could be related to a health condition.

- Your family history of mental and physical health.

From the referral stage, ADHD is handled differently, dependent on age. For children, watchful waiting is the first course of action before a referral is suggested. It is only after waiting that children will be referred to a specialist, and even then, group-based therapy and parent education classes are the preferred current frontline treatments for children with ADHD.

The reason for this is that doctors and psychologists are moving away from labeling to prevent limiting stigmas. Instead, they are opting to educate parents and children on how to overcome their weaknesses and work to their strengths. Whereas in the past, medicating children was the first line of defense against ADHD symptoms, now only the most severe and debilitating cases will be medicated.

Prescription medications need to be taken alongside therapy and education classes to give a child the best chance at managing their ADHD effectively and forming great habits to support success in adulthood.

For adults, however, the referral occurs earlier, and there is no true watchful waiting period. Your healthcare professional will use specific criteria to assess whether or not a referral is needed.

These criteria will include:

- Whether or not you had a previous ADHD diagnosis in childhood or slightly later.

- Whether or not you have been diagnosed with another mental health condition in the past.

- Whether or not your symptoms are affecting your day-to-day life. For example, are you underachieving in your job, or are your relationships suffering as a result of your symptoms?

In the past, the Diagnostic and Statistical Manual of Mental Disorders (DSM-5) was the gold standard for diagnosing mental health issues like ADHD. The DSM-5 is the standard diagnostic and classification manual used by healthcare professionals when identifying the symptoms and key traits of mental health disorders.

Lately, though, the medical and psychological fraternities have moved away from using DSM-5. The issue is that it perpetuates the notion that mental health disorders come with a genetic component when, in reality, 97% of these disorders have no known gene variants. Added to this, the DSM-5 insists that chemical imbalances are the cause of mental health disorders as a way to push pharmaceutical use (Ghaemi, 2018).

While I am not disputing that pharmaceuticals need to be used in some circumstances, there is no conclusive proof that medicine works for most mental health and behavioral disorders. The use of medications as a cure for mental health is 100% hypothetical, and pharmaceuticals are thought to mask symptoms rather than cure them.

Other issues with the DSM-5 include:

- a lack of scientific basis

- a disregard for other therapeutic methods that are based on science

- cultural bias

- a drive for pharmaceuticals as a "cure" for mental health

- the pathologizing of human experiences

- a label assigned to a person for life, limiting their experiences

As such, if you're seeing a physician for an ADHD diagnosis and have already received a previous one, you can expect a different experience.

The assessment phase of a diagnosis also varies from child to adult. A child may be referred to any one of the following specialists:

- a specialist child psychiatrist

- a pediatrician

- a child's ADHD healthcare professional

Adults will almost always be assessed by a psychiatrist and an ADHD healthcare professional. These ADHD healthcare professionals are usually general practitioners who have undergone additional training to understand the specific health needs of people with ADHD.

In most parts of the world, you can expect the following during your assessment:

- A physical exam to ascertain your general health and assert your primary healthcare physician's report on your health.

- A series of interviews with a psychiatrist, which may include different questions, exercises, and observations.

- A psychiatrist may also request to interview people who spend a lot of time with you, like your partner, friends, and family.

Once you have been thoroughly assessed, you will receive a diagnosis and a recommended treatment plan for your ADHD. Obtaining an ADHD diagnosis for a child is more difficult than for adults, as children must display more than six symptoms of attention deficit, hyperactivity, and impulsiveness.

Added to this, children must have symptoms for more than six months, have developed them prior to 12 years old, be symptomatic in different environments, and have a diminished quality of life due to their symptoms. Because of this, many children with ADHD are labeled as unruly when, in fact, they just don't fit all of the criteria listed.

Adults have fewer diagnostic criteria and usually have to show only five symptoms of attention deficit, hyperactivity, and impulsiveness. In addition, adults often have ADHD symptoms their whole lives, so they don't require a six-month waiting period.

Finally, it is a lot easier for adults to communicate that their symptoms are affecting their quality of life, which means symptoms only need to have a moderate effect on different areas of life.

These areas could include:

- underachieving in career or education

- reckless behavior with no explanation

- difficulties making or maintaining friendships

- difficulties regulating emotions

- relationship and familial difficulties

Current standards dictate that ADHD cannot develop in adulthood, and if your symptoms have only occurred later in life, there's likely another cause for what you're experiencing.

Childhood Symptoms

An inability to concentrate, hyperactive behaviors, and impulsivity are the hallmark symptoms of ADHD in both adults and children. It's important to remember that ADHD is a spectrum condition, which means you may have some symptoms working together to create an imbalance in your life, or you may be experiencing all of them.

In other words, you may find it difficult to concentrate but not be impulsive, particularly hyperactive, or you may be incredibly hyperactive and impulsive but can hyper-focus and concentrate pretty well.

Childhood ADHD usually presents with one or more of the following symptoms, which range from mild to severe:

- Uncontrollable fidgeting, wiggling, or foot tapping.

- An inability to stay seated even for short periods of time.

- An inability to wait—blurting out answers, pushing in lines, or shoving people aside.

- Outward displays of insatiable energy and a preference for running and climbing.

- An inability to remain quiet, even for short periods.

- A preference for gross motor skill activities over fine motor skill activities.

- Fine motor skills deficits.

- Excessive talking or talking for no reason.

- An inability to respect personal space.

Biologically, female children are more likely not to be diagnosed with ADHD, as symptoms and behaviors are more subtle but no less debilitating than those of their male counterparts.

Adulthood Symptoms

For most adults, hyperactivity is not an outward symptom of ADHD. This doesn't mean adults don't experience hyperactivity that they repress; it's just that it usually drives different behaviors than in kids, like emotional outbursts. For some adults with ADHD, poor coping mechanisms have been learned, and symptoms can present as other mental health issues, including perfectionism, defiance, or anger management issues.

In adults, symptoms of ADHD almost always co-occur, which means adults will have three or, most likely, all of the symptoms listed below:

- Feelings of restlessness or pent-up energy.

- Attention is focused on being calm and still, meaning they are unaware of other things happening.

- Impatience can result in emotional outbursts.

- Emotional dysregulation.

- An inability to allow others to finish their sentences or be quick to argue.

- Displays reckless behaviors without consideration for others at the moment but feels remorse afterward.

- Decreased tolerance for stress and frustration.

- Excessive talking.

- Can make inappropriate comments.

- An inability to complete tasks, sometimes seen as procrastination.

- Messy, untidy, and forgetful.

- Sometimes seems to be "operating" automatically.

- Anxiety and depression.

Brain fog, spacing out, being late, and feeling like mistakes are fatal can all compound anxiety and depression in adults with ADHD. Essentially, adult ADHD affects how well we can pay attention, whereas childhood ADHD affects how well we can train ourselves to pay attention. In childhood, ADHD presents ways to release pent-up energy, which is why kids with ADHD don't learn to concentrate and focus on the task at hand.

The Causes and Risk Factors of ADHD

To date, there has been no official conclusion as to the cause of ADHD. While some studies show there may be a genetic component, others can disprove this. The brain is a wonderfully complex organ, and there is still so much to learn about how it functions or what causes it to behave differently in people.

While parenting and the home environment definitely play some role in the behaviors a person learns, not all ADHD can be attributed to environmental factors. The nature versus nurture debate simply doesn't apply when it comes to neurodivergent conditions. A lot of the time, children can come from homes with no abuse or neglect, and a child may be diagnosed with ADHD or the like.

The fact that nature versus nurture doesn't apply to ADHD further compounds the question, "What causes ADHD?" Science is taking on this question by looking at the risks associated with the development of ADHD in children rather than trying to pin down any one underlying cause.

Brain Function or Anatomy that Is Altered or Different

Studies have been done to determine whether the way an ADHD brain functions is different from the way an average brain looks and operates. One such study focused on the brain activity of children and adults with ADHD. These studies revealed that people with ADHD have a frontal lobe that is different from people who do not have ADHD. The frontal lobe is responsible for our decision-making processes, voluntary movements, expressive language, and executive-level functioning. This study also showed differences in the arrangement of neurotransmitters, including noradrenaline and dopamine transmitters, the chemical messengers in the brain (Mayo Clinic, 2019).

Hereditary or Genetic Component

Research has both proven and disproven a genetic component in ADHD. However, new studies are investigating whether or not the condition may be caused by a combination of parental genetics or gene mutations (Balogh et al., n.d.).

Biological Gender

Statistics suggest that people who are born biological males are more likely to develop ADHD. It is theorized that hormonal and genetic factors may pose a risk when it comes to the development of ADHD.

Having said that, since boys are more likely to be impulsive and hyperactive, it's thought that girls are often not diagnosed. Treatment is never sought because girls are labeled as 'scatterbrained' or 'eccentric' as their symptoms present differently. It seems that the inability to concentrate and forgetfulness are the two symptoms both genders have in common, even in adulthood.

Fetal Exposure to Alcohol, Drugs, and Tobacco Smoke

Exposure to substances like alcohol, drugs, and tobacco smoke may be a risk factor for the development of ADHD in childhood. While studies do suggest a link between maternal health and well-being during pregnancy, nothing solid has been established, and no pathology has been discovered.

Again, most theories surrounding fetal exposure are hypothesized; however, it would appear that abuse of substances affects the nerve messengers within a fetus's brain. Added to this, exposure to environmental toxins may also be a contributing factor to neurotransmitter function and arrangement in people who do not have ADHD.

Exposure to Environmental Toxins in Childhood

In a world that seems to be filled with artificial flavors, preservatives, and sterile environments that coincide with the rise of ADHD in children, studies are being done into the effect of environmental toxins as a risk factor for ADHD. Lead exposure from paint and pipes has been shown to change behaviors in children, sometimes causing shorter attention spans and even violent outbursts (Donzelli et al., 2019).

Traumatic Brain Injury (TBI)

TBIs are injuries to the brain that are so severe that they alter the function of the brain. A TBI is caused by external forces like falls and accidents. Some studies show a small correlation between TBIs and the onset of ADHD in childhood, although none of these studies are definitive (Asarnow et al., 2021).

Foods Including Additives, Preservatives, Sugar, and Food Intolerances

While some foods that contain additives and preservatives have been shown to worsen the symptoms of ADHD, there is also some evidence that these chemicals could increase the risk of ADHD in children.

Refined sugars have also been linked with behavioral issues in children. Although studies have shown that there is no real association between sugar intake and the development of ADHD, sugar may escalate the symptoms of it.

In addition, children who suffer from food intolerances to common, healthy foods like milk, nuts, and wheat may be at an increased risk of developing ADHD due to the poor absorption of nutrition in the gut (Ryu et al., 2022).

Exposure to Television from a Young Age

There is some evidence that children who are exposed to long periods in front of the television may have an increased risk of developing ADHD. While studies on screen time are inconclusive, there is a correlation between screen time and attention deficits or the inability to sit still when the brain is not being actively stimulated (Stevens, 2006).

Intrauterine Growth Restriction (IUGR) and Premature Birth

Some studies show that babies born prior to 37 weeks of gestation, those born with low birth weight, or those diagnosed with IUGR are more likely to develop ADHD later in childhood. In addition, micro preemies (babies born extremely early and small) who suffer from brain bleeding at birth or after birth may have an increased risk of ADHD (Montagna et al., 2020).

As you can see, ADHD *could* be caused by a number of different things, but no conclusive or definitive proof has been discovered as to one specific risk or cause.

Common Misconceptions About Adult ADHD

Despite the amount of research and brain imaging findings that show ADHD results from neurological deficits or irregularities in the brain, ADHD is still massively stigmatized. When any condition is stigmatized, it comes with myths. These myths need to be dispelled to lift the guilt, shame, and sometimes blame that people carry around with them once they have been diagnosed.

Myth 1: ADHD Is Not a Disorder

This simply isn't true. Psychological, medical, and educational organizations all agree that ADHD is a legitimate medical condition. Where some confusion may come in is that certain institutions classify ADHD as a mental disorder, whereas others see it as a behavioral disorder. Regardless, ADHD is a medical condition that requires treatment to improve a person's quality of life.

Myth 2: ADHD Is Caused by Parenting

While upbringing and environmental factors do seem to play a small role in kids with ADHD, there is no conclusive proof that behavioral disorders are a result of a lack of discipline or parenting style. Even kids with overly strict parents may be diagnosed with ADHD, and may be more highly stigmatized by society because they are punished by their parent for behaviors they don't know how to manage.

Myth 3: ADHD Is a Male Condition

While it is true that more boys are diagnosed with ADHD than girls, gender does not play a part in how many people have ADHD. This myth persists because boys more often display disruptive, outward symptoms such as hyperactivity and disruptive behaviors that disrupt their classmates. In adults, men are more prone to have symptoms of risk-taking behavior and angry outbursts.

All of these symptoms mean males are more inclined to try to find a reason for their disruptive behaviors. On the other hand, females, who have more internally disruptive behaviors, are more likely to be diagnosed with a mood or personality disorder.

Myth 4: People with ADHD Cannot Be Successful

Again, this is absolutely not true. If history has taught us anything, it's that ADHD, when managed and channeled properly, doesn't need to be a hindrance, and anyone can be successful. In fact, some of the most influential and successful people of all time, including Mozart, Salvador Dali, Richard Branson, and George Bernard Shaw, all had or have ADHD.

Myth 5: Adult ADHD Doesn't Exist

There is a pretty common myth that children outgrow ADHD, and as

---

such, adult ADHD doesn't exist. The reality is that more than 70% of children with ADHD will continue to experience symptoms throughout their teen years, and about 50% will have ADHD in adulthood (Wilens & Spencer, 2010).

Now that you have a better understanding of ADHD and have dispelled some of the myths surrounding the condition, we can move on to how ADHD affects men specifically and the symptoms that drive our behaviors.

Chapter 2

Adult ADHD in Men

Anxiety does not empty tomorrow of its sorrows, but only empties today of its strength.

– Charles Spurgeon

Previous research suggested that ADHD does not affect males and females differently, and as such, mainstream treatments of ADHD were generic and did not focus on any specific set of symptoms.

Modern research, however, indicates that ADHD *does* affect biological males and females differently and that the type and severity of symptoms can differ between genders.

Psychiatry focuses on symptoms as a whole, which is probably why previous research suggested that ADHD presents the same way in males and females. In contrast, psychology focuses on shared human experiences rather than a set of symptoms.

Consequently, psychologists are at the forefront of changing attitudes regarding ADHD and how it affects males and females differently. For science to truly understand ADHD and create a system that is genuinely effective in managing its symptoms, there needs to be an acknowledgment that ADHD affects men and women in different ways.

How ADHD Differs in Men and Women

Before we explore how ADHD symptoms differ in men and women, we must take a look at how the frequency of a diagnosis can affect overall statistics and the reporting of symptoms.

Because boys are more likely to be diagnosed due to the disruptive symptoms they display, it can appear that males have an increased disposition toward developing ADHD. However, the reality is that the female symptoms are more introspective and less disruptive, meaning women are more likely to be misdiagnosed or completely overlooked when it comes to ADHD. This also means that females are less likely to receive medication or referrals to therapy, which would help them manage their symptoms.

Cultural attitudes toward boys and girls also influence how many children will be diagnosed with ADHD, as "boys will be boys" and "girls are eccentric and scatterbrained" biases continue to permeate our society.

In women, ADHD is also seemingly misdiagnosed more often than in men. This misdiagnosis could be because of female hormones, which play a role in fluctuating mood and altering brain chemistry throughout the course of the female reproductive cycle. It is thought that certain ADHD symptoms can be compounded by these hormones.

Regardless of a person's gender, an adult diagnosis of ADHD is far more complex than one in childhood. While there are fewer criteria to meet, healthcare professionals will have more comorbidities to consider before a diagnosis is given.

ADHD in Men

Men may present with some of the inattentive symptoms that women do, but generally speaking, men are more likely to have the outward disruptive symptoms of ADHD.

For males, the unique symptoms of ADHD are:

- outward hyperactive behavior

- disruptive displays of behavior

- forgetfulness and losing items

- interrupting

- outward displays of aggression

- participating in high-risk behaviors, including substance abuse and risky sexual behavior

- insensitivity toward others' emotions

While these symptoms are usually present in men, this doesn't mean that women don't sometimes have one or more of them. Having said that, men are far more likely to engage in these behaviors than women, and most men will have feelings of guilt and shame as a result of what they have done.

More common symptoms that can be experienced by both men and women include:

- difficulty sitting still or concentrating for long periods

- procrastination

- an inability to follow through with committed tasks

- not being able to manage time properly

- poor emotional regulation

- difficulty or inability to handle criticism or rejection

- an inability to identify risks or consequences

- difficulty putting their thoughts into words or actions

- frustration

- feelings of restlessness or wanting to fidget at all times

- an inability to follow a conversation or interrupt to change the course of a conversation

Intensity of Symptoms

What different scientific approaches do agree on is that the intensity of symptoms between men and women differs, although they haven't quite figured out why. The magnitude of hyperactivity seems to be far greater in males than in females, and the intensity of inattentiveness is more prevalent in females.

It is believed that the manifestations of symptoms often rely heavily on the societal roles people play due to their upbringing and the social environments they grow up in. This certainly seems to be true with men when it comes to relationship issues, risk-taking behaviors, and outwardly aggressive or disruptive behaviors.

We live in a world where it is okay for men to be aggressive or take risks, but it is not okay for them to speak about their feelings or be anxious. As a result, young boys with ADHD can grow into men who don't know how to manage or even identify their symptoms properly.

How the ADHD Brain Works

The ADHD brain doesn't only work differently from neurotypical brains; magnetic resonance imaging (MRI) shows that the development, function, and structure of ADHD brains are different.

These differences are what cause ADHD symptoms and the patterns of behavior that we form as a way of coping with our symptoms. For those of us with ADHD, our brain networks, size, and neurotransmitters don't function like other people's. Some areas of our brain can either over-function or under-function when they shouldn't.

A number of these differences may correct themselves or change from childhood through adolescence and finally into adulthood, which would account for the myth that people "grow out" of ADHD.

The reality is that the brain needs to be taught to change and how to function in certain ways. While it is possible for us to develop fresh neurons and neurotransmitters, we need to learn new things for these not to replicate themselves in their old forms.

In the past, it was thought that neuroplasticity, or the ability to create fresh neural pathways, was lost after adolescence. While it is true that kids learn new things a lot easier than adults due to the maturation processes in the brain, neuroplasticity is never lost. We can learn additional behaviors and information throughout our whole lives.

This means all is not lost when it comes to adult ADHD and is also why behavioral therapies like cognitive behavioral therapy (CBT) are so effective in helping to manage ADHD. For us to understand the ADHD brain, though, we first need to take a deeper look into how the function and structure of neurodiverse brains differ from neurotypical ones.

Functional Differences

The functioning of the brain is affected by ADHD in several ways that directly impact our cognitive, behavioral, and self-motivating processes. Added to this, certain types and intensities of ADHD may affect how well we regulate our emotions, feelings, and moods.

Emotions are a physiological function; everyone has them, and they're an evolutionary response we have developed to keep us safe. Emotions are fleeting and last around 90 seconds before fading away. Once we experience an emotion, we can decide to manage and eliminate it or prolong how we feel about it for a short while. Alternatively, we can choose to dwell on and stretch out these feelings, allowing them to affect our entire day, week, month, or even life!

Feelings and moods are choices; emotions are not. Anger can turn to irritation, and irritation can turn to, "My life is so hard, and everyone is against me!"

Because ADHD may affect how we respond to our emotions, it can also more dramatically affect our feelings and mood. We feel guilt or shame for our emotional outbursts and are unable to manage our emotions in the moment. For people with ADHD, the brain network is structurally altered, meaning it takes more time to develop. It also means it takes more effort to relay messages on what we should do with our emotions, behaviors, movement, focus, etc.

Added to this, certain regions of the ADHD brain can be either hyperactive or hypoactive, so no balance or regulation is happening in response to stimuli. The issue with only medicating ADHD is that we are never afforded the opportunity to correct our behaviors while consciously overriding the functional differences in our brains. This means we never learn the right coping mechanisms, nor do we stimulate the development of new neural pathways that will help us sustain fresh, positive behaviors.

Structural Differences

The ADHD brain has several structural differences when compared with neurotypical brains. Almost all of these differences can affect how a person behaves or reacts to their environment and the people they are interacting with.

These structural differences include a brain that is slightly smaller than neurotypical ones, with slower maturation rates, and volume differences in the amygdala and hippocampus areas of the brain. It's important to know that brain structure doesn't affect intelligence in the least, only the ability to process information at what society deems to be a 'normal rate.'

Structural differences in the brain may affect how well we regulate our emotions and recall memories from our subconscious and our level of self-motivation. The frontal cortex, which is responsible for our ability to concentrate, plan, and perform other cognitive functions, is most affected by maturation differences. This could be why restlessness and fidgeting will increase, and time management will be affected when we have ADHD.

The motor cortex, which controls movement in the body, is often more mature in people with ADHD, which is why kids with ADHD usually do really well in sports if they are allowed to focus on these skills.

These structural and functional differences in the brain are what define ADHD as a behavioral and not a mental health condition. And this brings us full circle to the DSM-5, which deals with mental disorders.

In addition, these differences in the ADHD brain suggest that the condition should be treated based on behavioral and mindset changes, with medical assistance where needed. ADHD cannot be medicated away, but yes, medication may be needed to help some people function. However, you need to be willing to work on your behavior, practice self-love and acceptance as you rehearse your new skills, and take action every day. This will help your brain rewire itself so that you can manage your symptoms more effectively.

Common Challenges Men With ADHD Face

Men with ADHD face specific challenges that are mainly unique to them. While I don't want to stereotype any one gender, it's important to know which challenges are most specific to men with ADHD, so you know what behaviors you should be working on.

If you tied your shoelaces wrong your whole life and the laces came undone, frustrated you, and caused you to fall and hurt yourself or others, wouldn't you want to know that you were tying them wrong?

Psychologists who work with men with ADHD have identified certain patterns of behavior that impact their quality of life and that of the people they are friends or in relationships with. These commonalities are pretty vast, but the most typical of them are listed below.

Career and Work

For many men, their identity is wrapped up in their profession and ability to provide the lifestyle they think they deserve. While there is nothing wrong with basing some of your identity on your job, it can become an issue for men with ADHD, as behaviors that are not addressed can cause problems at work.

Many men with ADHD find that they are fired from their dream jobs, constantly on the edge of disciplinary action, or isolated from their peers, which creates an unpleasant work environment.

A lot of these outcomes are consequences of ADHD behavior that has not been addressed. Not finishing tasks, having to be micromanaged to get work done, emotional outbursts, and interrupting people in meetings or while they talk can all negatively compound over time.

Other ADHD symptoms that can affect work are:

- forgetfulness

- impulsivity

- poor timekeeping

- disorganization

Often, men with ADHD also display some form of defiance, as their ego seeks to protect them from feeling shame and guilt for their behaviors. This defiance is often the driving factor behind men with ADHD being fired. This pressure to achieve goals can lead to slacking off work, which is directly interpreted by leaders as willful misconduct or non-compliance.

Time Management

Distraction, fixation, forgetfulness, and the inability to anticipate the consequences of actions can all lead to poor time management and procrastination, ultimately resulting in productivity becoming static.

Men with ADHD are not natural planners and, as such, have issues with deadlines. As more and more tasks pile up, defiance and defensive behaviors can begin to be used as a shield against why tasks haven't been completed.

Because ADHD is a behavioral condition that affects our executive functions, we can tend to live too much in the present and not enough in the future. This means we have a hard time understanding what the rewards are for getting a task done, preferring to fill our lives with instant gratification.

This tendency can cause issues for us as our friends and partners become frustrated with us for being constantly late or not following through with our commitments. Of course, it also affects work performance, as procrastination often means failing to achieve the goals set for us.

Disorganization and Clutter

Some people with ADHD do well with clutter and disorganization, while others can get lost in the mess they have created. It can sometimes be difficult to figure out whether or not the clutter and disorganization created are causing more harm than good.

Here's a good measure of whether you are organized or not. If your controlled chaos wastes time while you look for things, slows down your ability to get tasks done, or creates an unhygienic environment, it's no longer organized. Disorganization and clutter are hallmarks of ADHD that follow most children into adulthood.

Some kids learn how to deal well with chaos and disorganization. When they become adults, this disorganization brings them comfort and actually increases their ability to get tasks done. However, others are swallowed up by their disorganization, which affects everything from their job to their relationships. A good benchmark for assessing whether clutter and disorganization are beneficial to you is to ask, "Is this costing me time?"

Risk-Taking

When we take risks, adrenaline is released into our bodies, and this hormone surge can also signal our brains to release dopamine. Because the neurons that respond to dopamine are often not fully mature in people with ADHD, more dopamine is needed for them to feel the effects of being happy or content. As such, people with ADHD may take risks so that they can increase their feelings of well-being.

Risk-taking behavior can be further compounded by not fully understanding or thinking about the consequences of their actions, which can lead to impulsive and reckless actions. It's important to note that risk-taking behavior can range from minor to severe. Being late for events, interrupting conversations, or picking petty fights with your partner may all be part of your risk-taking behavior.

Severe risk-taking behaviors like driving dangerously or too fast, abusing substances, infidelity, and committing crimes are usually escalations of minor risks taken at a younger age. If you are participating in severe risk-taking behavior, this is something that needs to be addressed by a medical professional as soon as possible. There are much safer and healthier ways for people to balance dopamine production and uptake that should be discussed with a healthcare professional as a matter of urgency.

Sleep

While poor sleep is often not listed as one of the symptoms of ADHD, men specifically say that their sleep is incredibly poor as a result of the condition. The reasons for bad sleep range from having too many thoughts whirling around to rumination, restlessness, too much energy, or overstimulation. In fact, more than 80% of men with ADHD report having trouble falling asleep and staying asleep at night (Pera, 2022).

Sexual Infidelity

Many men value their performance in the bedroom and use their sexual performance as a key influencer of how high or low their self-esteem is. Having ADHD can affect sexual performance by making it harder for a man to please his partner. This leads to feelings of failure and ultimately drives the need to improve their self-esteem through other means.

When risk-taking behavior and impulsivity are brought into the equation, men with ADHD may begin to develop poor habits that destroy relationships. Online pornography, strip clubs, extramarital affairs or cheating, and engaging in unprotected sex all come with very serious consequences that men with ADHD often don't think about.

Afterward, however, these consequences can become very real, and anxiety and depression can threaten to overcome a person, leading to suicidal ideation. Studies show that men with ADHD who are not actively working on their behaviors are 50% more likely to participate in sexually risky behavior and infidelity (Sarkis, 2011).

Less Treatment

Men are taught from a young age that the behaviors surrounding ADHD are "guy things" and that what they're experiencing is normal, which could not be further from the truth. As a result, many men with ADHD will never seek treatment, nor will they speak about how the challenges they're facing are causing them emotional hurt and harm.

In addition, the stigma surrounding mental health and the misplaced perception that ADHD is a mental health disorder can mean men are more likely to suffer in silence when it comes to ADHD. Of course, this compounds many of the issues men face when dealing with ADHD. Ultimately, a man can lead himself to believe that it is just his "lot" in life: to suffer instead of thrive. ADHD is not a condition that corrects itself.

While many men have learned adequate or even great coping mechanisms for dealing with the symptoms of ADHD, there are a whole lot more who are genuinely suffering needlessly.

ADHD Men in Relationships

Men with ADHD can present with two extremes when dealing with relationship conflict. They can become very easily annoyed and animated in their irritation and anger, or they can become conflict-avoidant, which develops passive-aggressive behaviors. Both extremes can be very detrimental to personal and romantic relationships, negatively impacting the person with ADHD and those on the receiving end.

Additionally, romantic relationships can become strained due to a lack of attention to detail, messiness, and having to be constantly reminded to do small tasks. Significant others may feel like they're being neglected or that their role has shifted from a life partner to a parental role as they are constantly managing their ADHD man's behaviors and mess.

When relationship troubles begin to arise for ADHD men, they may have difficulty expressing what it is they're going through or how they feel. In turn, this can be extremely frustrating for their partners.

Up to 70% of men with ADHD suffer from emotional dysregulation that can cause angry outbursts, often directed at unsuspecting partners (Beheshti et al., 2020). Emotional dysregulation can also create a dopamine feedback loop in which ADHD men seek out conflict behavior as a way to stimulate brain activity.

For ADHD men in relationships, this can create a negative behavior pattern. A calm and peaceful relationship is replaced with a game of drama and problem creation so that they can build excitement and feel better temporarily.

Of course, this is highly detrimental to any relationship as it erodes intimacy and creates a toxic relationship environment. As a result of emotional dysregulation and the creation of problems, many men with ADHD are wrongly labeled as narcissists.

While having ADHD doesn't excuse abusive behavior, knowing why you may be creating a problem in your relationship can help you fix the very behaviors eroding your intimate connection with your partner.

ADHD Comorbidities

ADHD changes a person's life, and receiving a positive diagnosis gives them an opportunity to improve their quality of life. Whether through medication, therapy, or a combination of these two treatment options, alongside dietary changes, exercise, and a willingness to change, ADHD can be very effectively managed.

While most people with ADHD may need to fine-tune their treatment plan until they're doing well in their lives, others may find that no matter how hard they work, they're still battling with their ADHD. The reason for this is not ADHD itself but the fact that almost half of all people with ADHD have a comorbid condition (Silver, 2023). Comorbid means that more than one condition is occurring simultaneously.

Comorbid conditions that affect men with ADHD include:

- anxiety

- depression

- obsessive-compulsive disorder (OCD)

- oppositional defiant disorder (ODD)

- difficulties learning

- gross and fine motor skills difficulties

- executive function difficulties

- tic disorders

Most of the time, these disorders are the primary cause of the symptoms of ADHD, and as such, only co-occurring symptoms of both conditions will get better with treatment. Other times, secondary disorders are triggered by prolonged exposure to ADHD symptoms. For example, a person may suffer from chronic anxiety as a result of not being able to perform due to their anxiety. Alternatively, someone may develop depression because they feel guilt, shame, or fear that they will not succeed in life. A person is usually diagnosed with a comorbid condition when the symptoms of ADHD are not sufficiently resolved with treatment.

Generally speaking, there are three ADHD comorbidity categories:

1. Cortical wiring disabilities include learning, language, fine and gross motor, and executive functioning difficulties.

   These comorbid conditions can be rectified with proper lifestyle changes and behavioral therapy; they do not usually require medication.

2. Emotional regulation disabilities include depression, anxiety, anger control, OCD, ODD, and bipolar disorder.

   These conditions require professional medical intervention and medication to help correct chemical imbalances in the brain and body. ADHD is usually a secondary condition to these, and medications need to be properly prescribed and monitored by a psychiatrist or physician.

3. Tic disorders that include motor and oral tics, as well as Tourette's syndrome, are disabilities that are not common but can occur due to certain ADHD medications.

Throat clearing and physical tics are typical side effects of medicines like methylphenidate (Ritalin and Concerta) and mixed amphetamine salts (Adderall and Mydayis).

A healthcare professional will lower the dose of these ADHD medications or stop treatment altogether to see if tic symptoms improve. If they do not, a comorbid condition will be diagnosed.

The Strengths of ADHD and How to Use Them to Your Advantage

So much emphasis is placed on ADHD as a disorder or a weakness. The reality is that with every weakness comes strength. It is the law of nature that everything created must have balance for it to work effectively. It is our weaknesses that make us unique, and our strengths allow us to balance out the things that don't work all that well for us.

Even neurotypical people have weaknesses. The difference is that people who do not have a diagnosis for a condition or disorder don't usually focus on their deficiencies. To harness our strengths, we need to do the same: Focus on what makes us unique and tap into our ADHD superpowers to help us overcome our weaknesses. When we learn to tap into our strengths while working on our weaknesses, we can turn our ADHD into a formidable ally that drives our success.

ADHD Hyperfocus

Not everyone has the ability to hyperfocus on tasks without ever having to take a break, and even fewer people can tune out the world to immerse themselves in what they are doing.

For people with ADHD, hyperfocus usually occurs when they are doing something they find really interesting, enjoying themselves, or have set their minds to completing a task. With ADHD hyperfocus, task completion can be used to improve productivity, work more efficiently, and outperform neurotypical people. Fewer distractions also mean that the quality of what is produced in a hyperfocused state is often far better than other neurotypical people's work.

Resilience

A growth mindset, in which we believe we can achieve anything we set our mind to, requires resilience. Without resilience, we can give up too easily or spend too much time analyzing why things aren't working rather than noting why our task failed and then trying again.

People with ADHD have had to overcome many obstacles in life, facing rejection and failure more often than neurotypical people. As such, those with ADHD are far more likely to be resilient to difficulties. Setbacks and adversity are a part of life for people who are neurodivergent, and when resilience is tapped into, just about any obstacle can be overcome.

Ridding ourselves of a "victim mentality" and choosing to use our ADHD in our favor will help us tap into our resilience and ensure we can work past our setbacks efficiently. Additionally, resilience builds a strong mental character that other people look to for guidance and inspiration.

Some of the best leaders and most successful entrepreneurs, like Richard Branson and Ingvar Kamprad (the founder of Ikea), have received an ADHD diagnosis. However, these people didn't dwell on their weaknesses, instead choosing to work within their strengths and resilience.

The trick with resilience is to become deeply self-aware of our behavior to know when we're the cause of the issues around us and when something is happening to us. When we become self-aware, we can identify what needs to be worked on and take the necessary steps toward success.

Creativity

One of the hallmark strengths of ADHD is creativity and the ability to approach goal-oriented tasks from a different perspective than neurotypical people. Having ADHD and living with it throughout childhood requires finding alternative solutions to the common issues and problems life can present. This different approach means people with ADHD inherently become amazing problem-solvers and can often come up with multiple solutions to one issue.

Impactful Conversational Skills

Most boys with ADHD will be described as excessively talkative, and this trait is often carried through to adulthood. However, because men with ADHD have learned over time what is acceptable in conversation and what is not, they have fine-tuned their conversational skills. Additionally, as people with ADHD are creative and take on problems differently from others, their conversations are often interesting and engaging.

While men with ADHD may have lower emotional intelligence, they have a much higher level of social intelligence in comparison with their neurotypical counterparts. All of this means those with ADHD have the ability to become profoundly impactful masters of speech and can use this skill to make a difference in the world.

Courage

People with ADHD have to overcome a lot in their lives so they can live peacefully with self-love and acceptance. Along with building resilience, courage is a byproduct of overcoming these challenges. Over time, learning courage and the ability to ascertain the difference between good and bad risks can help men with ADHD become highly sought-after employees.

Instead of overthinking situations, people with ADHD who have learned to assess risk quickly will make a decision and work through any obstacles resulting from that choice.

Boundless Energy

Another one of the hallmark traits of men with ADHD is a lot of energy. Whether this energy is internalized or not is irrelevant, and when men can learn to use this energy constructively, they can often outperform their colleagues at work.

This energy is also why so many men with ADHD excel in sports and other recreational activities. When creating a balance between focus and ways to burn off this energy in a constructive way, men with ADHD can truly use their superpowers to their advantage. The trick with ADHD is to stop focusing on the weaknesses the condition presents and start looking at all of the amazing strengths it has to offer.

For many people, ADHD has been the greatest gift they have received because they have learned to use their neurodiverse brains to their advantage. Like other conditions, ADHD is only disabling if you allow it to be. It's important to remember that ADHD does not define you; *you* define how you will use it to your advantage.

How to Overcome the Stigma and Shame of ADHD

I'm sure people have told you that there is absolutely nothing wrong with receiving an ADHD diagnosis. Yet these words often don't come with comfort as societal stigmas continue circulating, leading to deep feelings of fear, guilt, and shame.

We can begin to think that we are flawed and weak rather than seeing all we have overcome to get to this point in our lives. Feeling shame about being diagnosed with ADHD is counterproductive as it highlights perceived weaknesses instead of strengths.

Receiving your ADHD diagnosis is a blessing. It lets you know that your unique brain can be used to your advantage and helps you specifically identify weaknesses that you can work on. However, if you are battling with your diagnosis, here are some ways you can overcome the stigma and shame that accompany ADHD.

Find a Mentor or Read About Other ADHD Men's Successes

Believe it or not, thousands of people around the world have received an ADHD diagnosis, and many of these people are incredibly successful. Instead of focusing on all the negative things people are saying, it's important that you also seek out success stories. That way, you can not only find the commonalities in any symptoms you may be experiencing but also see how other people used these symptoms to their advantage.

Seeking out someone who can mentor you is also a great way to help you identify where you may be battling and uncover areas of strength. A mentor with ADHD will also allow you to relate better to their struggles and form a bond with someone equally unique.

Surrounding yourself with information and educating yourself on other people's successes will also help you understand that ADHD doesn't mean you're broken. You're just different, and uniqueness is a sought-after trait.

When you do have moments of feeling low, remind yourself that some of the greatest and most creative minds in history used their ADHD to entertain, educate, and invent, making others' lives better and happier.

Set Aside the Victim Mentality

I know it's a harsh realization, but everyone has their own struggles, some smaller than yours and others much larger. Going through struggles is part of life, and without setting aside your victim mentality, you'll never be able to see your strengths or utilize them to your advantage. With tenacity, knowledge, and an embrace of your diagnosis, you could potentially be unstoppable.

When You Feel Weak, Highlight Your Strengths

No one denies that ADHD comes with frustrations and weaknesses, but it also comes with many strengths you can take advantage of. It's important to understand that when it is channeled properly, ADHD can be your greatest strength, and it can actually accelerate your journey to achieving your goals. Of course, there will be days when you feel frustrated and down because you're battling against yourself, but in these moments, it's a good idea to remind yourself of all your other strengths.

Be Accountable

Once you have received your diagnosis, you're presented with a choice: To become responsible for your own future and health and be accountable for your actions, or to live the rest of your life using your ADHD as an excuse for your behaviors.

For anyone to overcome stigma and take control of their lives, they first need to acknowledge that a problem exists and then look for solutions to this problem.

Is your journey to success going to be perfect?

No!

Are you going to stumble and make mistakes along the way, slipping into old habits from time to time?

Yes!

But this doesn't mean you're not responsible for being accountable when it comes to your own journey in life. Becoming accountable for your actions and life will mean you spend less time on things that are not productive for your future and more time on improving your life. You will begin to understand the impact your actions have on others. You will also start to value everything you have overcome while celebrating all the milestones you have achieved so far.

Once you become accountable, your confidence will begin to soar as you realize that stigmas mean nothing if you pay no attention to them. Finally, overcoming the stigma of ADHD requires you to step outside of a negative mindset and embrace all the positive things the world has to offer. You need to be able to work on your own thoughts before you can change other people's outlooks on what ADHD is and how it affects those who have it.

Working on your thoughts and ensuring that you are developing effective coping mechanisms, building your self-esteem, and practicing emotional intelligence will change your actions, and actions always speak louder than words. Over time, you will begin to prove to yourself that your ADHD is less of a disability and more of a superpower that you have been blessed with.

Your ADHD is absolutely not a curse, nor is it a disease that you need to feel any guilt or shame for. You have the same, if not more, opportunities to succeed as so many other people. It all begins with how you choose to manage your thoughts.

Chapter 3

Your Thought Spiral

You don't have to control your thoughts; you just have to stop letting them control you.

– Dan Millman

Overthinking isn't necessarily a bad thing. Everyone has moments where they may overthink a situation before taking action, but it can become an issue and potentially create a much larger problem for you.

Being stuck in our thoughts is a symptom of ADHD, drawing our time and attention into scenarios that may or may not be true. Overthinking traps us in a never-ending spiral, repeating the same thought and applying it to different situations without any end goal or aim.

Under normal circumstances, overthinking can be halted by consciously choosing another topic and switching to it so that you can move on. In the ADHD brain, though, changing to a new topic can have you applying the old topic to the new one, forcing you to process the same thought over and over again in every situation.

Being stuck in a thought spiral is detrimental to our mental health, not only because it takes up our time, but also because it can, over time, begin to be the root cause of depression and frustration.

Unfortunately, ruminating thoughts are also a metaphorical magnet in our brain, pulling in one bad memory after the next and driving us to relive everything negative that has happened in our lives.

Because the ADHD brain works differently from the neurotypical brain and certain areas of the brain can be overly active, overthinking can be a symptom of the condition. When overthinking persists and a person allows rumination to overtake their life, comorbid conditions like OCD can occur.

The Side Effects of Overthinking and ADHD

Overthinking can come with a lot of unpleasant side effects; some, like depression and losing time, have already been discussed. Almost all of the side effects of overthinking are not great, and the five most common of these are listed below.

1. **We begin to isolate ourselves from people**: Rumination can make us believe that people don't like us or that our ADHD is a burden to others. As a result, we begin to remove ourselves from society. Over-discussing every situation and conversation we have is exhausting, to say the least, so instead of putting ourselves through that, we start to feel that it would be better if we were alone.

    Additionally, when we ruminate, we may perceive other people's actions or words as hurtful without considering their intent or empathizing with what they are going through. Instead, we lash out and become hurtful, forcing others to stay away from us.

2. **We begin to lose confidence**: A lot of the time, when we ruminate, our thoughts aren't about what others have done but about what *we* have done. We start to focus on our mistakes, leading us to lose confidence in our abilities. Replaying our mistakes repeatedly, even if we only made this mistake once, can make us feel like we've made an endless number of mistakes when, in reality, we're just as imperfect as the next person.

3. **Our body begins to react physically**: When stress levels go up, our mental and physical health takes a beating. Subjecting our minds to stressful thoughts and reliving these stressful moments creates a situation in which our body remains in a stress response. Being stuck in this stress response increases blood pressure and heart rate and lowers our immune system.

4. **We begin to hyper-focus on things that aren't constructive**: Yes, hyper-focusing can be one of our greatest strengths. However, when our attention is focused on negative activities, like ruminating thoughts, we start to lose time and disrupt everything from our productivity to our sleep patterns. Managing hyper-focused behaviors is near impossible if we're stuck in a thought spiral that is affecting our mindset.

5. **We run the risk of developing analysis paralysis**: The term 'analysis paralysis' is when we can't make decisions or feel stuck in our own lives due to overthinking a problem. While analysis paralysis may not seem to be rooted in fear or negativity, it is often a result of us reliving our mistakes or fearing the outcome of the decisions we make.

Consequently, instead of making a decision, we begin to analyze all possible and sometimes impossible variables, being stuck in a loop of imaginable solutions rather than taking action.

Calming the ADHD brain can sometimes feel like an impossible task, especially when it is trapped in a thought spiral that threatens to consume us. Developing healthy strategies to help manage our overthinking tendencies and make meaningful decisions for our present and future is vital to our success and mitigating the risk of developing comorbid conditions.

Strategies for Managing Your Overthinking Tendencies

You already know that overthinking is normal and that even neurotypical people will have moments when they overthink their circumstances. For the ADHD brain, changing thought processes or distracting ourselves may sometimes work, but generally speaking, snapping out of a thought spiral requires us to have solid strategies in place. When we don't manage our overthinking tendencies, we can drive ourselves into anxiety and depression, not only compounding our negative thoughts but also intensifying our other ADHD symptoms.

It's difficult for those of us with ADHD to acknowledge that most of the time, the problem isn't what *made* us ruminate but our persistence in ruminating. We must take into account that our brains have a natural tendency to hyperfixate and that certain areas of them are hardwired to be overactive or underactive. Therefore, thought spirals that aren't managed with proper strategies can really harm our mental and physical well-being.

Strategies such as stepping outside of our thoughts or challenging our feelings may work very effectively. However, the fact of the matter is that most people with ADHD simply haven't been taught how to use these strategies specifically for their minds. For example, if I told you to sit quietly and clear your mind for mindful meditation, how long would you be able to do this before fidgeting, boredom, and finally, your thoughts reentered your mind? You need to be able to take the techniques that work and apply them to your life and your unique brain so that they effectively manage your thought spirals.

Mindfulness Meditation for ADHD

For men with ADHD, internalized symptoms of boundless energy can lead to frustration and, ultimately, emotional, angry outbursts. Paying attention and practicing self-regulation can feel impossible when you need to fidget or move constantly. Self-regulating our behaviors and emotions is something we need to fine-tune and hone for the sake of our job and our relationships. Learning how to do this is one of the most invaluable tools anyone with ADHD can learn.

Most people know that mindfulness meditation is a powerful self-focus practice that has been around for centuries. Nevertheless, there are many misconceptions about the process that can turn those with ADHD away from it. The first and most common of these misconceptions is that you need to sit quietly and clear your mind in order for mindfulness meditation to work. This is simply not true!

Mindfulness meditation can be done at any time and in any quiet place for as little as five minutes, and you really don't need to clear your mind at all. The entire point of mindfulness is to observe your thoughts without judgment, letting them pass by without giving them attention or further analysis. As you begin to hone your mindfulness meditation skills, you start learning how to focus your attention on your emotional state or surroundings without feeling the need to react.

Another misconception is that you can practice mindfulness meditation a couple of times and feel a marked improvement in your ADHD symptoms. Again, this is not true because the nature of mindfulness meditation is to build a tolerance for a new behavior over time.

Think of mindfulness meditation as learning to swim. Most of us don't just jump into the deep end and expect to know how to swim like a pro. In fact, most people don't even expect to float! Like swimming, you need to wade into the shallow end and teach yourself how to focus your attention over time, eventually reaping the rewards of the practice.

Research shows that 15 minutes of mindfulness meditation per day improves mood, concentration, and emotional regulation, which contributes toward a much higher level of mental well-being (Alhawatmeh et al., 2022).

Cognitive Behavioral Therapy (CBT) to Help Curb Overthinking

CBT is an evidence-based type of psychology used to identify our negative, biased thoughts that influence our behaviors. Once a thought is identified, CBT teaches us how to reframe these thoughts and properly deal with our anxieties in a way that benefits us.

Thought spirals and overthinking are almost always based on cognitive errors, which means our spirals are caused by thoughts that are not true. Thought spirals and cognitive errors are not unique to people with ADHD; in fact, everyone has them!

The difference between a neurodiverse and a neurotypical brain is how these cognitive errors are processed. For most neurotypical people, cognitive errors will be challenged. The truth about the thought will be ascertained before disregarding the information the brain has presented the person with.

The neurodiverse brain, however, will often begin to fixate on these cognitive distortions, trying to find solutions to the false information it has provided. This creates a loop, or spiral, in which the neurodiverse person will repeatedly play the same thought scenario in their head while they try to find a solution to something that doesn't actually exist.

I'm not saying all neurotypical brains work this way. Some people will experience thought spirals without having ADHD. The issue with thought spirals is that they cause a lot of anxiety, which can develop into depression. Here's the good news, though. CBT is a proven way to help deal with these cognitive errors, breaking thought spirals and improving mood, concentration, and sleep.

The Triple-Column Method

This CBT exercise, created by David Burns, is the most effective way to challenge cognitive errors and help prevent thought spirals before they begin or stop them when they start. Studies conducted on the triple-column method show that when combined with conventional talk therapy, this exercise is extremely helpful in helping regulate emotions, manage stress, and regain control of our thought patterns (Belmont, 2017).

Of course, the first step in regaining control of your thoughts is to identify your cognitive distortions by journaling your thoughts as they happen. Any thought that isn't factually true or that you wouldn't say out loud to someone else is most likely a distortion.

There are several different kinds of cognitive distortion. Here are descriptions and examples of the most common ones:

- **All-or-nothing thinking:** Seeing things as black and white with nothing in between. *I will never be good enough.*

- **Blaming (Personalization):** Feeling responsible for everything that happens. *My colleague was rude to me today. I must have upset them somehow.*

- **Catastrophizing:** Blowing things out of proportion and thinking the worst will happen. *My boss has asked to meet with me tomorrow. I think I'm going to be in trouble and get fired.*

- **Emotional reasoning:** Believing your feelings truly relate to reality. *I feel like a total idiot, so I must be one.*

- **Fortune-telling:** Believing you can predict future outcomes. *They are offering a promotion at work. I'm sure one of my colleagues will get it instead of me.*

- **Ignoring the positive:** Focusing on any negatives in a situation, regardless of your success. *I got a thank you email from my boss today, but I bet he's sending them to everyone.*

- **Labeling:** Applying negative labels to yourself and others. *I am such an outcast here; everyone else thinks they are so amazing.*

- **Mental filter:** Picking on a negative thing and letting it affect your feelings and actions. *I know most people said my presentation was good, but I got a couple of feedback sheets that told me how to improve it, so I feel like it went really badly.*

- **Mind-reading:** Assuming you know what other people are thinking. *One of my colleagues didn't talk to me this morning. They must be upset about something.*

- **Overgeneralizing:** Taking an event and/or behavior and thinking it will happen consistently in the future. *I am always late, and I always make people angry.*

- **Shoulds & Musts:** Commanding yourself to do things. *I should be on time. I must leave the house 30 minutes earlier every day.*

Now that you know how to identify your cognitive distortion and the different types of distortion, you can create your triple-column exercise:

1. Grab a blank piece of paper, your journal, or create a new Excel spreadsheet.

2. Divide this blank page into three columns. Try to make sure you have a couple of new, pre-prepared pages so that you have your three columns handy when a thought spiral begins.

3. Label your columns as follows: column 1—Automatic thought; column 2—Distortion; and column 3—Rational response.

4. Trigger warning! Seeing your thoughts in print is often shocking and may make you sad or angry. Try to push through this stage.

5. When you have a negative thought, write it in the automatic column.

6. Now, write what the distortion is. Why is this thought untrue?

7. Next, write down the rational response to the thought.

Here's an example.

- **Automatic thought**: "I am the worst partner! My girlfriend or boyfriend hates me, and they're only with me because they feel trapped."

- Read your thoughts and say them out loud.

- **Distortion**: Overgeneralizing and getting into an all-or-nothing thought process. Mind-reading what my partner thinks without getting their feedback. Catastrophizing my relationship.

- **Rational response**: "I could probably do better in my relationship; everyone should try to be a better partner today than they were yesterday. My partner tells me and shows me that they love me often. There is no actual evidence that my partner wants to leave me or that they feel trapped in the relationship."

You can write down or type out as many of your automatic thoughts as you want, so don't limit yourself. At some point, your brain is going to get tired of being challenged. It will shut down your thought spiral, replacing these thoughts with confidence-boosting positive thoughts.

Like mindfulness meditation, this exercise will not work overnight; it takes time to be able to catch yourself at the beginning of the spiral and identify your distortions.

You need to become comfortable with not only recognizing when your brain is trying to hijack you, but also identifying the thoughts you are having that are exaggerated or simply not true.

If you find that you're battling to identify your thoughts or if you're becoming really frustrated with yourself during the process, take a break. Remove yourself from the situation, and take five minutes to meditate.

Like everything else in life, it takes time and practice to hone your skills, but you're at a distinct advantage, so tap into your ADHD brain's superpowers and use your tenacity and perseverance.

Part 2

Self-Regulation for Positive Transformation

Chapter 4

Your Guide to Mind Mapping

It is not easy to make things simple - one must be sufficiently disgusted with brainless complexity.

– Dharmendra Rai

Mind mapping is a technique with several uses, including brainstorming. It doesn't require too much thought about structure and visualizes ideas so that strategies can be made to put them into action. When we are mind mapping, we essentially create a visual representation of tasks, concepts, emotions, and even the words we want to express without these elements having to be linear or organized.

In other words, mind mapping allows you to turn an abundance of thoughts into a diagram. It helps you to be organized so that you know what steps need to be taken to achieve an end goal or objective.

The best thing about mind mapping is that it is an external representation of how the human brain naturally works. This makes it perfect for people with ADHD, especially when important concepts need to be discussed or when simply creating an organized method of getting things done.

Neurodiverse and neurotypical people alike can benefit from creating mind maps as they can process information faster and recall important information much more easily than having to sift through all their daily thoughts.

In a day-to-day setting, mind mapping is used to:

- visualize concepts and brainstorm ideas

- communicate ideas so that they can be presented

- create an organizer for tasks that need completion

- run meetings in a more organic, engaging way

- summarize documentation and reports

- simplify thought processes, tasks, and projects

- communicate thoughts or emotions with more accuracy

Mind mapping is designed to help you discover what hidden strengths lie in the recesses of your subconscious mind by allowing you to put your thoughts on paper. With regular practice, it can be an incredibly powerful tool for becoming productive at work and at home. But where did the mind mapping concept originate from?

Dr. Roger Sperry, a Nobel Prize winner for his research, began studying the human brain in the early 1900s. During the course of his analysis, Sperry discovered that the cerebral cortex was divided into two hemispheres and that each hemisphere was responsible for a range of tasks.

These tasks include recognizing color, daydreaming, imagination, logic, rhythm, distinguishing lines, lists, and words, and the ability to see the bigger picture. What Sperry ascertained throughout his research was that these activities are all integrated. The higher the number of these activities being done at the same time, the more effectively the brain works to stimulate the intellect and achieve objectives.

The result of this research was mind mapping: A way in which people could exercise all of the fundamental areas of the cerebral cortex to maximize information processing and use their brain's full range of cortical abilities.

Mind mapping uses many of the functions of both the left and right hemispheres of the cerebral cortex. Therefore, people with ADHD can tap into the power of their brains to clarify, organize, and structure their thought processes without the risk of running into a negative thought spiral or bad hyperfixation.

How Mind Maps Work

Now that we know what a mind map is, we can explore how it works and why it is such a valuable way of retaining and recalling information. A mind map is the most creative and logical way of translating environmental stimuli and information into a comprehensive plan your brain can use to become more productive.

Answering the question, "How do mind maps work?" is simple. It's the creation of a detailed roadmap to where the brain stores information. Here's an example.

If a friend had moved home and you were due to visit them, they would provide you with clear, concise directions to their new home using road names and landmarks. They may even send you the coordinates of their new home so you can use GPS/ an app to show the route to your destination.

By looking at the map, you can check you're going the right way by identifying the landmarks your friend mentioned. When driving there, you will follow the directions provided by your GPS/app or by your friend to arrive at their house.

If the instructions were clear enough, using words and lines in the form of directions (left, right, and straight), and you had visual cues such as landmarks to let you know you were going in the right direction, your brain will use this information to get you to your end goal.

Mind mapping works in the same manner, and by using natural organizational structures, lines, and visual cues, your brain can be trained to reach an end goal or objective in a much easier way. Let's go back to the map example.

Over time and the more often you visit your friend, the more familiar your brain will become with recalling the landmarks and directions you initially provided it with. Eventually, you'll be able to drive to your friend's home without any instruction or active thought processes.

The end goal of mind mapping is to train your brain to filter thoughts in a way that allows you to place them on paper. Then you can use the information that is needed and disregard any that is not required.

Ultimately, you will learn how to assimilate and use information quickly and without much thought.

Before I get into how to create a mind map and some techniques you can use to help you become a mind mapping ADHD master, let's look at the key elements of an effective mind map.

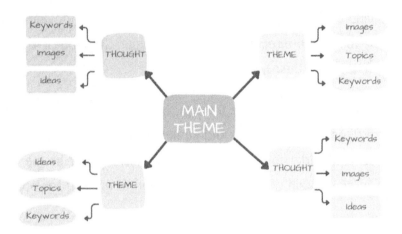

- Every mind map must have a central focus point. This can be a subject, a focus point, or a main theme. You can even use an image for this main theme if your mind works better with imagery than words.

- Lines must be used to connect themes or thoughts to the central main theme. These lines are called branches.

- Each branch must have a keyword or image placed at the end of it.

- Each branch can have topics, keywords, or images in the form of a line that is not that important to the central main theme. These lines are called twigs.

- Every branch must be relevant to and connected to the central theme, but not every twig has to connect to the central theme, only to a branch.

A Step-By-Step Guide to the Mind Mapping Process

Mind maps can be created on paper or digitally, and there are a number of great apps, which will be mentioned later, available to help people create seamless maps. Regardless of your mode of creation, mind mapping needs to follow a specific process and set of steps for it to be effective.

The Main Theme

This will be the central focus of your mind map and is the reason, purpose, or the *why* behind your map. All mind maps start from the middle and branch outward, so the central idea must be the core topic of your map.

Here are some ideas for why you might want to create a mind map:

- You're facing an obstacle or challenge that you're unable to work through, e.g., you want to find a new job.

- You're brainstorming ways in which you can become more organized and productive at work.

- You're battling to grasp a difficult concept or idea.

- You're trying to simplify a complex idea or piece of information.

- You're trying to break through a creative block.

- You would like to express complex emotions or feelings.

- You would like to set attainable goals for yourself.

Add Your Branches

Once you have your central theme, you can begin your map by adding branches to cover subtopics. These branches don't need to be organized in any way, shape, or form and shouldn't contain much information. Keywords and short phrases are more than enough information for you to create a proper branch.

If your mind wanders while you are creating your branches, add a twig and place this information on the twig if it doesn't deserve its own branch. These branches will be the source of information for your center point.

Add Twigs

Once you have branches attached to your main theme, you can begin to add twigs to each branch. The only rule with twigs is to ensure the information you are adding is relevant to the branch. If it isn't, then it shouldn't be on your mind map, and you can disregard the thought.

There is absolutely no limit to the number of branches or twigs you can add to your mind map. Thus, let your brain wander, and see how many thoughts and ideas you can come up with that pertain to your central theme.

Add Some Colors and Images

Just like your roadmap to your friend's house, the information on your mind map will be better stored and more effective if you add landmarks or visual representations of where you should be in your journey.

Adding colors, shapes, and images will also ensure you are engaging both lobes of your cerebral cortex, thereby maximizing your brain's ability to process and store information. The more areas of your brain you use when creating your mind map, the more likely your brain will be to retain the information and recall it later on.

Here is a working example of a mind map when planning how to find a job. This main theme is placed in the center.

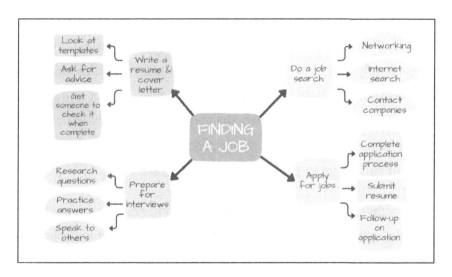

Branching off from the main theme are four topics that are steps in the process of finding a job. Moving around the map in a clockwise direction, starting with the top left box, these are: write a resume and cover letter; do a job search; apply for jobs, and prepare for interviews.

These branches then separate off into twigs that show the relevant and connected tasks that need to be done. For example, when writing a resume and cover letter, it is worth doing some online research and looking at templates. You may know other people who have recently done this, so you can get some advice, and when you have completed these documents, you can ask them to check for any mistakes or missing information.

Mind Mapping Techniques for Men With ADHD

The world of business has never moved faster than it does today, and ADHD can sometimes be a distinct disadvantage for men in the workplace. Disorganization, procrastination, and taking longer to do tasks can all hinder productivity within the workplace. This can subsequently lead to feelings of inadequacy, frustration, and sometimes disciplinary action from management for not completing tasks. For men with ADHD, job satisfaction and a work-life balance can be challenging as productivity slips and personal relationships begin to suffer due to pent-up energy and stress.

Both partners in a relationship generally work, so they are expected to assist with household tasks to help split the mental and physical load within the home. Mind mapping offers men in the workplace a unique opportunity to organize their home and career spaces, becoming more organized and efficient with the tasks that need to be done in both places.

All of this leads to a greater sense of accomplishment, self-confidence, and the ability to shine in professional and personal roles. While the basics of mind mapping remain the same, the techniques of mind mapping for men with ADHD may require some tweaking for the tool to be completely effective.

The reason for this is that most adult men with ADHD have a lifetime of dysfunctional habits they have learned. While these habits can be unlearned, it takes time, effort, and the right tools, plus the ability to be productive and efficient in the moment.

With all of this in mind, it's important to remember that the basics of mind mapping will remain the same. There must be a main theme in the center of the page. Branches come from it with ideas, information, or interconnected concepts, and wings break off into additional ideas. Each of these ideas must be interrelated; if other themes crop up, a separate mind map can be created for each of them.

The difference between standard or neurotypical mind maps and ADHD mind maps is simplifying or disseminating the information on the mind map. As the ADHD brain is generally far "busier" than the typical one and because some irrelevant information may be transferred onto a mind map, it's essential to refine it.

Additionally, a mind map should be used to create a concise list of milestones or objectives that break tasks down into smaller, more manageable ones to achieve a greater goal.

Here's how to refine your mind map:

- Identify your central theme as usual.

- Add details in the form of branches and twigs, as usual.

- Look for relationships between your central theme and your branches and twigs.

- Separate these relationships by color. Choose your own colors or use red for branch themes, black for dates, blue for explanations, green for facts, and another color for additional information.

- Once you have your twigs and branches color-organized, begin looking for your organizing principle. This principle is the logical sequence in which your tasks should be done. For example, you wouldn't hand in a task you haven't completed yet, or put the vacuum cleaner away if you haven't yet vacuumed the house. This step may take some time when you first start mind mapping, but it will get easier with time.

- Move your tasks around in chronological or logical order. Place your central theme at the top of your list. Use your colors to discern whether your tasks are, in fact, in the right order. Run this order through your mind or say it out loud so that you can double-check that it makes sense.

  Any branches or twigs that are not yet on your chronological list will need to be checked to see whether they need to be a part of your process. Slot them into your list where they need to go or discard them if they are not required.

- Finally, redraw your map with your items in chronological order. In this final draft, look for ways to make your objectives and milestones stand out. Use colorful borders, images, or other visual reminders to help prompt you with the next steps you should take.

- Put your finalized mind map up where you can see it and consult it when you need to do a task. Once you have completed a task or an objective, be sure to tick it off your map and celebrate your victory in achieving this milestone.

You should find a non-material way to reward yourself whenever you get a task done or complete one of your objectives. It is a critical step in creating new habits to replace your dysfunctional ones. This is because habits are formed in a loop that involves a routine, a cue, and a reward. In creating your own routine, cue, and reward cycle, you'll be effectively developing a habit loop that benefits your life and well-being.

Mind Mapping Tools and Technology

One of the greatest things about living in a modern technological era is that technology can help us simplify, organize, and visualize our thoughts and ideas, allowing us to have a clear mind map to success. Mind mapping tools and software enable us to give structure and order to our complex ideas, connecting all the steps we need to take to achieve a goal.

Mind mapping software is an amazing way to simplify the process of creating a mind map for whatever purpose you need. This may include making changes to your personal life, bringing your vision boards to life, and becoming more productive at work.

The benefits of using mind mapping tools and technology include:

- The simplification of your mind mapping process and creation:

Mind mapping software and tools allow you to create a comprehensive list of ideas and thoughts in one space that color codes your projects as you develop. Modifications to this thought process don't require you to create a whole new mind map, as changes can be easily applied digitally.

- The ability to collaborate with other team or family members: Collaboration ensures you are not working at cross-purposes with the people in your life. Collaborative maps that allow invited members to contribute their ideas are extremely helpful in creating behaviors that facilitate great interpersonal relationships.

- The integration of other apps: Being able to integrate other apps into your mind mapping process is incredibly valuable, especially in the early phases when you may need reminders to begin tasks. Integration with programs such as Google Workspaces, calendars, and Microsoft Teams means you'll never miss a reminder or opportunity to share your progress and the planning of your day, as well as facilitate great collaboration.

- Software creates mind maps that are easy to follow: While traditional mind maps are great, their format may not work with each unique brain. Using mind mapping tools and technology will give you a choice of how you want your map to be displayed. You can select the way that best resonates with your brain, creating an effective memory jog and call to action. In addition, mind mapping tools will allow you to add different elements to your map, and you can customize everything from your line styling to your colors and even your branch and twig positioning.

Now that you know the advantages of using mind mapping tools and technology, you can begin to explore the various options available to you.

Suggested Mind Mapping Technologies

Below is a list of some of the more popular mind mapping tools available across different platforms. This is by no means an extensive list, and a quick Google search will provide you with many tools for your specific mind mapping purpose:

- **MindGenius**: A simple-to-use tool that includes customizable backgrounds, branch shapes and fills, and custom task boards that allow you to track your milestones.

- **MindMeister**: A great collaborative mind map that lets you share your ideas, milestones, and goals with other people. The app is cross-platform, which means it can be used and accessed across browsers and devices such as Android and iOS.

- **Xmind**: Features minimalist interfaces and simplistic charts and layouts for people who don't like busy mind maps. Each layout is customizable, and the software includes logic charts, brace maps, tree charts, timelines, etc. The software is cross-platform for browsers on Android and iOS.

- **SimpleMind**: For people who are not technologically advanced, SimpleMind is straightforward and easy to use. It offers different templates and forms of mind mapping that include monthly planners, flowcharts, and organizational charts.

These are only suggestions for the different software options available to you. It's up to you to find a mind mapping tool that works best for you and your specific needs. Remember, everyone's brain works uniquely, and this means different tools and software will not resonate the same way for everyone.

Incorporating Mind Mapping for Workplace Productivity

You now know that mind mapping can be an incredibly effective tool for helping you build your organizational skills and become more productive. Since men with ADHD often face battles in the workplace, mind mapping can be used as a way to become a valuable member of your company's team. Mind mapping in the workplace can range from creating basic maps to using more complex and specific forms of tools that can help build and maintain focus.

The most common of these mind maps are listed below. Have a look at each of these, do some further research, and try to use whichever applies to your role or position in your company.

Flowcharts

The most basic form of mind mapping in any organization is done with flowcharts. They use mapping symbols and illustrations to display the inputs and outputs of a process, plus each specific step and milestone required to achieve a goal.

Basic flowcharts are usually used to plan projects, document processes, improve communication, brainstorm solutions, and manage workflows. Flowcharts are the best tool to show how a project will progress from start to finish.

High-Level Process Maps

These mind maps show a process from the top down, which gives a much higher-level view of a goal. These mind maps only show the essential steps in achieving a goal and, as such, contain only minimal details.

Generally speaking, high-level process maps are solely used to define business processes and identify the key areas required to achieve success. High-level process maps are used to illustrate and discuss processes with a third party that isn't actively involved in a specific project.

Detailed Process Map

Detailed process maps are the exact opposite of high-level process maps and specify each process and sub-process required to complete a task. The hallmark of this type of mind map is that it documents each decision point as well as the inputs and outputs needed for each step of a project. Detailed process maps are the most effective way to create a visual understanding of complex tasks, identifying areas of possible inefficiency and how to overcome them. Detailed process maps are best used to develop an understanding of a process and to list contingency plans.

Swimlane Map

This mind map is cross-functional and is sometimes called a deployment flowchart. The goal of a swimlane map is to designate certain activities for people. Each of these activities is situated in a swimlane.

Every swimlane is assigned to a specific stakeholder who will be responsible for the activities within that channel. As such, swimlane maps are great for new employees who don't know their roles or processes properly yet, or to increase accountability within a team.

Value Stream Map

This type of mind map is primarily used as a lean management tool that assists in the visualization of the processes required to create a product or service. Value stream maps are very complex, using specific symbols rather than words to help illustrate the flow of the processes as well as any materials required.

While documenting this data may not seem like a big deal, value stream data allows teams and external stakeholders to identify when products and materials need to be delivered. This saves valuable time during a project as less time is focused on what is happening or needs to be acquired next. It allows each person to focus on what is required of them right now.

As such, value stream maps are best for highlighting the processes involved in developing a product or service and documenting each process with quantitative data.

SIPOC Diagram or Map

SIPOC stands for suppliers, inputs, processes, outputs, and customers. While SIPOC diagrams are not really maps, they do chart certain elements of a process that are key to success. Usually, SIPOC diagrams are used as a precursory step in drafting a more detailed process map for a team or individual.

SIPOC diagrams are presented with a minimum of five columns. In each of these columns, the processes, outputs, and inputs of the process are highlighted, as well as any other pertinent information.

This type of map is used to prepare detailed process maps by defining the scope of more detailed or complex processes. It also identifies key elements and the stakeholders involved in a process from start to finish.

Symbols You May Need to Know

Mind maps that are used in the workplace will often come with specific symbols. These symbols are called Unified Modeling Language (UML), and each of them represents the elements of a process, including inputs, outputs, steps, decision points, and stakeholders.

Each organization that uses mind maps will train its team members in this language and the symbols associated with it. In the meantime, here is a list so that you can begin your corporate mind mapping journey:

- **Oval:** Denotes a terminator, which is the beginning or end of a process.

- **Rectangle:** Denotes a step, activity, or task involved in the process.

- **Arrow:** Denotes the directional flow of the steps in the process.

- **Diamond:** Denotes a decision and will be displayed when a critical decision needs to be made. These will be answered yes or no, and branches will be given for both responses.

- **D:** Denotes a delay.

- **Parallelogram:** Denotes data that is part of the input or output of the process.

- **Rectangle with a slanted top:** Denotes data that needs to be manually entered.

- **Rectangle with double vertical lines:** Denotes a subprocess that doesn't necessarily directly pertain to the project but is needed.

Tracking Your Progress and Achievements

Once you have created your mind map, the next phase is to institute the steps you have created for yourself. Actioning your mind map will ensure you are making steady progress toward achieving your goals. Plus, it's also important to actively track your progress so you can celebrate your successes and achievements.

Before reading the steps below, I'd like you to know that there is no metric or measure for success because everyone's definition of success is different. Getting up in the morning, leaving your home neat and tidy after doing five minutes of mindfulness meditation, and arriving on time wherever you're going is a success.

Successes and achievements can sometimes be the minuscule things we do that facilitate a better life, great habits, and overall well-being. You simply cannot impose someone else's definition of success on yourself. You can absolutely look to others for inspiration and ideas but always remember that this is your life, which means applying the things that are important to you.

Take the time to define success for yourself and decide what small changes you need to make so that you can ultimately reach your end goal. Now that you know what success looks like for you and what you'd like to improve and work toward, let's get down to how you can track your progress.

- Break your achievement goal into milestones. You may know what you want to achieve, but you'll need to create steps for how to get there. Mind mapping allows you to create these milestones so you can list them in order of priority. The goal here is not to change everything at once but one small thing at a time.

- Set deadlines for your milestones, not your goal. It's best not to set a deadline for your actual goal but rather to set completion dates for each milestone, deciding when you will have accomplished or instituted each of them. In setting timeframes for your milestones, you are not overwhelming yourself with the bigger picture. It's the old analogy of how to eat an elephant ... one bite at a time.

- Tick off your milestones and celebrate them! That's right; you need to focus on rewarding yourself for the small actions and steps you're taking. This is because your goal will be self-rewarding, but if you don't celebrate each milestone achieved, it's going to begin to feel like you're running a never-ending marathon. Celebrate all of your success, but more specifically, celebrate your consistent improvements.

- Consider turning your mind map into specific, measurable, achievable, relevant, time-based goals (SMART). There is a reason SMART goals work: they're broken down into smaller milestones with deadlines that can be monitored and tracked with precision. SMART goals automatically create a map that is specific, measures your progress, and ensures you can move toward your end goal in a sustainable way.

- Review where you were and where you are. A great way to celebrate your small victories is to look back and see how much you have progressed over a short period of time. Reviewing your progress and even documenting it if you like will help you remain motivated when it feels a little overwhelming or like you're not doing enough to progress. It's normal to beat yourself up on bad days, but it's also important that, in those moments, you acknowledge your progress too.

If you feel like you're losing track of your progress or have lost sight of the bigger picture altogether, you're not alone. Many people come across obstacles as they put their mind maps into practice.

Some of these common obstacles include:

- Fixating on the details rather than taking action.

- Getting too involved in the type or aesthetic of the mind map.

- Not organizing the information gathered from the mind map.

- Not combining your mind maps to ascertain common goals or purposes.

- Not using images and colors that resonate with you or only using words.

- Not summarizing your thought processes or being too long-winded with your map.

Always remember that your mind map is a way to focus your thoughts into a clear, concise plan that should be used to improve your life and achieve your goals.

Be thoughtful in the creation of your mind map, avoid common mistakes, and understand that the definition of success is extremely personal. This will help you take the steps you need to take in your own journey to achieving your goals.

Chapter 5

Executive Functioning 101

If you want to be happy, set a goal that commands your thoughts, liberates your energy, and inspires your hopes.

– Andrew Carnegie

Executive function skills and the ability to self-regulate go hand-in-hand. Without executive functioning, we are unable to remain focused, follow instructions, or complete multi-step tasks effectively. Consequently, if we do not learn executive functioning, our brain cannot prioritize tasks, control our impulses, set or achieve goals, or filter out environmental distractions.

Human beings are not born with executive function skills. They are developed throughout childhood and adolescence via exposure to other people, correction, and life experiences.

Children and adults with executive dysfunction can struggle in life as the positive behaviors expected of them to integrate into society and make good choices are lacking.

Additionally, children who don't learn executive functioning skills also lack self-regulation, memory, mental flexibility, and self-control skills. Therefore, they experience more challenges than typical children.

While this may not sound like a major problem, the reality is that executive function skills are highly interrelated with other neural functions, including working memory, mental flexibility, and the ability to control impulses.

It's important to note that although no one is born with executive functioning skills, everyone has the ability to develop them. Children with neurodiverse brains may just require a little extra support in developing these skills. Sadly, most children with ADHD are not afforded this support because neurotypical adults find ADHD difficult to manage.

They are placed in traditional classrooms, where teachers are often assigned more students than they can cope with; therefore, children with ADHD do not receive individual attention for developing these skills. This creates a compounded issue in which children grow up without the very skills they need to belong in society.

While more attention has been brought to ADHD as a real behavioral condition in modern society, entire generations have grown up without these critical skills, creating a group of adults who are seriously struggling through life.

Children and adults with ADHD need to be in environments that promote growth. They need to practice these critical skills safely so they can begin to establish the right routines and start to model good social behaviors.

Developing an understanding of executive functioning, practicing the required skills, and learning to manage stress effectively all contribute toward fast-tracking proper neural function.

A Deeper Understanding of Executive Functioning Skills

Executive functioning is a set of skills that include your memory, the ability to control your impulses, and being flexible in your thinking. These skills are used every day of our lives to manage tasks at work and at home, to create a sense of belonging in society, and to regulate our emotions.

With executive dysfunction, it can become very difficult to follow instructions, focus on anything, recall memories or information, and regulate your emotions effectively. All of this contributes to stress, lowered self-esteem, and a feeling that you don't belong in society.

While I have briefly explained what executive function is, it is important that you have a deeper understanding of it and how it directly affects your life. This understanding will serve as your purpose or the *why* behind learning these critical skills, and will be addressed in a later chapter.

A great way to think of your brain is that it's a busy international airport. There are multiple flights landing and taking off 24 hours a day, passengers rushing to get to their gate or to be picked up, people sitting about in restaurants, and others trying to catch up on their work tasks for the day.

Without air traffic control, information desks, and proper signage, the airport would be chaotic. No one would know what was expected of them, where they should go, or when they were expected to get onto a plane that may or may not be able to take off or land safely.

Airports need management systems for them to run safely and correctly, and so does your brain. This neural management system is executive function, and it ensures working memory, cognitive flexibility, and inhibitory control are in place.

Without executive function skills, attention span, organization, planning, prioritizing, task completion, the ability to see different points of view, emotional regulation, and self-monitoring are all lacking. Neurotypical brains will learn executive functioning skills as a part of the normal social correction process, but they can continue to develop well into a person's 20s. A lack of special attention to these skills in neurodiverse people can mean they lag behind their typical peers and, as a result, have more challenges when they are adults.

Some of the primary signs that you are a neurodiverse person who is lacking in executive skills include:

- Struggling to begin or complete tasks.

- An inability or battle to prioritize tasks.

- Having poor short-term memory or forgetting things you've heard or read.

- Struggling to follow sequential steps or directions.

- Needing a routine or panicking when a routine is changed.

- Struggling to switch focus from one thing to the next.

- Becoming fixated on things.

- Having an emotional response to situations or struggles that are not a big deal.

- Struggling to focus or organize thoughts.

- An inability to manage time.

An ADHD diagnosis means that there is an executive function issue, but when these critical skills are not developed, other comorbid conditions like learning disabilities can arise. Having said that, people can have executive functioning issues without having ADHD, and people can think differently or struggle with certain aspects of these skills without having any disorders. Not having the right grounding in executive functioning skills does not mean a person is stupid, lazy, or belligerent.

What Causes Executive Dysfunction?

Research into what causes executive function issues is still pretty new, but preliminary findings suggest there are two main contributing factors. When reading this section, you should keep in mind that people with ADHD will always have some level of executive dysfunction, especially if special attention and skills-building have not been a part of their treatment plan.

The reason people with ADHD have executive dysfunction is rooted in neural differences. Men with ADHD are more likely to carry executive dysfunction into adulthood because hyperactive behaviors and a lack of concentration are labeled as hallmark male traits.

The two main reasons for executive dysfunction are:

1. A brain that is neurodiverse, which causes certain areas of the brain to be under or overactive.

Certain areas of the ADHD brain develop differently from neurotypical ones, and the ones used for executive skills like memory and emotional centers may evolve more slowly.

While science is not sure why this happens, genetics may play a role, and people with executive dysfunction may find that family members suffer from these dysfunctions too.

2. Environmental factors may contribute to executive dysfunction. These may include having a parent with executive dysfunction, not having a proper emotional attachment to parents, abuse, economic hardship, neglectful caregiving, and chaotic home environments.

Some studies suggest a third possible cause is that learning disorders may be a factor in executing functional challenges. Having said that, research has neither proved nor disproved this, so these findings are purely opinion-based at this stage.

Executive Dysfunction Diagnosis

There are no official diagnostic criteria for executive function challenges. Regardless, during the review and assessment process for an ADHD diagnosis, executive function will be assessed.

Some of these assessment criteria will include:

- the ability to maintain attention

- inhibitory control

- issues with short-term memory or working memory

- issues with planning or organization

- concept formation issues

- inability to move from one task to another easily

- word and idea generation issues

Testing for executive functioning challenges will almost always be done as part of a full evaluation for other comorbid conditions. It's important to go to a licensed, registered mental health professional like a psychologist or psychiatrist when testing executive functioning.

Boosting Executive Functioning

People with ADHD have issues with focusing their attention, hyperactivity, and impulse control, which can lead to executive dysfunction. Deficits in executive function can lead to a lowered sense of well-being and cause practical issues in a person's professional and personal life.

Because everything from cognitive skills to planning and prioritizing is affected by executive dysfunction, other comorbid conditions can begin to surface, and the most common of these are anxiety and depression.

For people who are medicated for their ADHD, executive functioning does not improve. Studies show that as many as 80% of people who are medicated for their ADHD will have no improvement in their ability to focus, short-term memory function, or distractibility without actively working on these skills (Roth & Saykin, 2004).

Medicating ADHD without addressing or correcting the behaviors associated with the condition and without teaching the skills required to improve executive function is like placing a bandage on an infected wound.

Issues need to be addressed from the inside out so that new neural pathways can be formed and the development of good habits can begin. In his Psychology Today blog, Scott S. Shapiro, M.D. describes five strategies that can be used to help improve executive function skills in relation to adult ADHD and work.

Step 1: Clarify Expectations

The first step in developing executive function is to clarify what needs to be done, how it should be done, and by when. Men with ADHD are often extremely enthusiastic about setting and achieving goals but lose momentum quickly. The reason for this is that goals and expectations are often not well-thought-out or time-bound and lack clear direction.

Having clear expectations often goes beyond personal goal-setting. In a workplace where the ADHD man is expected to perform well and achieve milestones, not having clarity can lead to hyperfixation or confusion. The ADHD man's enthusiasm for tasks, while helpful, tends to stall achieving goals as they don't have an understanding of or clarity on the steps required to complete these milestones and goals.

To negate this issue, it's important that questions are asked and the answers are written down.

Here are some questions you can ask to help guide you in setting expectations.

1. What is the goal, and what does success specifically look like?

2. What is the time frame for each milestone required for success?

3. What is the scope of this project?

4. What specific details should be paid attention to for this project to be a success?

It's important to ask as many questions as you can to gain clarity on what is expected of you.

Step 2: Request Feedback

Men with ADHD can tend to view failure as something fatal or a reflection of their character. These thought distortions often stem from early childhood when their behavior provoked angry responses from adults or other kids ostracized them. Thought distortions can instill a deep sense of self-doubt, shame, and avoidance of doing tasks for fear of failing or making a mistake.

Asking for regular feedback or creating a positive feedback loop is a great way to know that you are on track with a project and meeting all the required expectations.

Organizations will often insist that leaders meet with their staff on a monthly basis. However, more regular feedback meetings are hugely beneficial to people with ADHD so they can remain on track with their assigned tasks.

Meeting frequently with leaders and stakeholders also instills a sense of accountability and improves motivation. It also allows changes to be made during the process rather than waiting until the end of a project when issues may become overwhelming or irreversible.

Step 3: Write Out Strategies

The nature of modern workplaces is that teams often undertake large projects, so every team member must pull their weight to complete the project successfully. This can potentially cause issues when strategies and expectations are not clear, which can lead to people with ADHD feeling isolated or that they have let other people down.

An easy way to overcome this is to make sure strategies are written out in a simplified format, showing each milestone and the steps that need to be taken to achieve them.

Mind mapping is a great way to do this, as it enables men with ADHD to visualize a project properly and effectively without becoming overwhelmed with everything that needs to be done.

There are other ways to write out projects in the form of flowcharts, as discussed in the previous chapter, and the simple steps that can be taken to achieve an end goal. The ADHD brain works best when it is offered a combination of visual and physical stimuli, which is why handwritten strategies are preferred over typed-out ones. Studies show that writing notes activates more areas of the brain and leads to better recall of the information.

If you would prefer to use an app, that's fine, but do write out your strategy before transferring it to your app. Handwritten strategies don't need to be super precise or perfect by any means, but they should anticipate all of the steps required or the questions that need to be asked to remain on track with a goal.

Step 4: Add Tasks and Milestones to a Calendar

For most people, calendars with proper reminder notifications are useful, but for the ADHD brain, they're a necessity. Most men who have overcome executive function issues will tell you, "If it's not documented with reminders set, it simply doesn't exist!" When critical tasks are not recorded in a diary or added to a calendar, there is a big chance that they will be forgotten about or fall through the cracks.

This means listing all of the steps of a project with their deadline dates and setting reminders that allow adequate time to get the milestones done. When adding reminders, you're ensuring nothing slips by unnoticed and putting a contingency in place that helps you stay informed about upcoming tasks. It's a good idea to both write these steps out on paper and add them to an electronic calendar so that visual and kinetic stimuli come into play.

Step 5: Create an Organizer's Handbook

Men with ADHD can sometimes be oblivious to socially acceptable behavior or the rules of engagement in an organizational setting. This is by no means intentional, but once awareness is brought to this conflicting behavior, it should be changed quickly to prevent social isolation.

Creating an organizer handbook filled with the rules, regulations, and expectations required to be a functional member of any team is the perfect ADHD tool for building executive skills.

This handbook can contain information on people that will help you bond with them. You can log anything outside of project scopes that need to be done by you, organizational requirements or rules you tend to forget, and feedback you have received that will help you improve. Think of your handbook as a "master guide."

Having this kind of instruction manual allows you to enter social and professional situations armed with knowledge. It removes the fear associated with feeling or acting differently or letting people down.

Time Management Strategies for Men With ADHD

The restless and impulsive nature of people with ADHD can create time blindness because they think of time differently than neurotypical people. These time perception differences can also mean people with ADHD have issues estimating how long tasks will take, how much time needs to be spent on each milestone, and when tasks should be done.

Research has shown that ADHD distorts time in the brain because it requires a number of sections, including the prefrontal cortex, anterior cingulate, and supplementary motor area (Weissenberger et al., 2021).

This means deadlines and showing up on time are a real struggle for people with ADHD. However, procrastination, improper planning, and becoming distracted easily are all manageable symptoms.

Take a look at the strategies below. While they all work, it's up to you to try each of them and implement the ones that help you manage your time more effectively.

Externalize Your Time

People with ADHD can struggle to understand time as a whole concept, so it's important that you question time to gain proper clarity.

Questions like:

- What is this due, and by when?

- How long should this task take? Can you please be specific about a date and time?

- How well have I managed my time so far?

Asking questions like these helps supplement the brain's internal ability to process time, but these internal reminders may be forgotten without externalized tools like clocks, calendars, or audible reminders.

For the ADHD brain, analog clocks are best to help process time properly, and they can help the brain become consciously aware of the passage of time. Successfully managing time begins with awareness of time and intentionally acting within prespecified boundaries.

In other words, even if you're aware of what the time is and you can see the clock moving, the chances are you won't pay attention to it unless you have a reminder or alarm that pushes you to take action.

If you are one of those people who is a stickler for details or are stuck in a rut of procrastination, setting high-priority reminders will help you take action more effectively. Proactive time management ensures you will be able to complete more tasks and accomplish more during the day. Nevertheless, you should be aware of overfilling your schedule with too much in a day.

It's normal to become enthusiastic about your newfound time management skills, but it's important that you don't overdo it. Block out your time and ensure you prioritize the tasks that have to be done before the things you *want* to do.

Practice Essentialism

American author and business strategist Greg McKeown coined the term 'essentialism' as a way to decide in what areas a person would like to succeed in their lives. The reality is that everyone can't be good at everything all the time, nor do they have to be. By stopping trying to do everything and focusing on what is essential, people can achieve their goals faster and contribute more to the world.

To implement an essentialist lifestyle, you need to define what it means to succeed and, more specifically, what success means to you. That way, you can deliberately allocate your precious time and energy to the things that matter. When you are in control and can choose the things that are important to you, you're creating value and reward in your actions.

Considering your strengths, decide what tasks have to be prioritized, including those chores we all hate doing if they cannot be delegated to someone else. Then make a list of the things that are important to you and that you believe will bring value to your life. Use these things as a way to experiment with your time management and be progressive in taking the right action to achieve your goals.

Learn to Time Block

Looking at the bigger picture and seeing everything that needs to be done can feel overwhelming. Time blocking allows you to focus your attention on one chunk of a task at a time, with the understanding that completing smaller quantities of a task will get everything done on time. For example, you might block out two 30-minute time slots in your calendar each day to respond to emails rather than being distracted by them as they arrive.

Time blocking also lets you celebrate the smaller milestones you have accomplished, leading to higher motivation toward completing the full task. How you block out your time is entirely up to you, and the only prerequisite to time-blocking is to ensure that critical or priority tasks are completed first. In Chapter 7, there is a practical exercise to do to get you started.

Keep To-Do Lists Updated

A master list is an amazing organizational tool, but it can all amount to nothing if you are not keeping your lists up-to-date and crossing off completed items.

Having a to-do list is also a great way to preserve your energy and attention because you're not trying to remember all the important things that need to be done on a day-to-day basis.

With any to-do list, consistency is key, and if you are one of those people who has a lot to do, create more than one master list so that the crucial tasks for the day in each category can be tackled first.

Having more than one master list will also show you whether or not you've overcommitted yourself and allow you the opportunity to delegate tasks that are not critical for you to do.

Finally, don't get too caught up in things you shouldn't be doing. Instead, focus on what *must* be done and then tackle the items you want to do once these critical tasks are complete.

Make Use of Tech

Technology can serve as one of our greatest distractions or one of the most effective tools we own to help manage our time. Every smartphone can be used to set reminders, create task lists, and have a calendar with notification functions. Visual and audio reminders are an amazing way to help keep you aware of the time and when to shift to the next task.

Analyze Your Brain's Patterns

Everyone has times when they are most productive or when it feels like everything works seamlessly. Conversely, there are certain periods of the day when we can become unproductive for no particular reason. If we're not careful about managing them, these unproductive times can threaten to derail our entire day.

Analyzing your brain's productivity patterns will allow you to schedule your concentration-intense tasks during your effective times and use your less productive periods to complete tasks that don't require your full attention.

Rather than focusing on the periods you are battling to concentrate or beating yourself up about struggling through tasks, reshuffle your day and time-blocked segments to help your brain work when it's at its optimum.

The more you analyze your brain's patterns throughout the day, the more opportunity you give yourself to work efficiently and productively. In addition, by allowing your brain time to rest while still being productive on non-intensive tasks when concentration levels are low, you're building a sense of achievement *and* ticking things off your to-do list.

Create Routines Around Your Patterns

The brain remembers things more easily when it has a routine because routines are patterns too. In fact, your brain will respond to these routines better if you split them into daytime and nighttime routines.

The trick to creating a routine is to work around patterns you have already formed for your life. For example, if you brush your teeth after drinking your coffee in the morning and take your medication while you pick up your car keys, it's important that you don't disrupt this pattern. Instead, you could add something to your routine in slow or "dead" moments. What do I mean?

Let's say you have ten free minutes between drinking your coffee and brushing your teeth. You fill this time with scrolling social media before heading to the bathroom to continue your routine.

If you broke these ten minutes in half, you would have five minutes to practice mindfulness meditation and five minutes to scroll social media without disrupting your routine. In fact, you would've created a pattern within a pattern if you consistently practiced your mindfulness meditation every morning, building upon your habitual patterns.

Routines developed around our brain's patterns help us function more efficiently and ensure we're not wasting time, which ultimately makes us feel terrible. Analyzing our behavioral patterns also allows us to see how much time we're spending doing things that are not healthy or productive for us so that we can make better choices.

Gift Yourself Time

Ask anyone with ADHD what causes them anxiety, and somewhere on their list will be rushing from one thing to the next. Rushing around or knowing that you're going to be late or won't have enough time to complete a task will cause you to feel stressed out, even if you aren't consciously aware of your stress.

This anxiety and being late for things are inevitable, especially when your brain simply doesn't perceive time in the same way as a neurotypical one. A fantastic way to overcome this issue is to gift yourself time by allowing yourself a grace period between tasks or when having to leave to go somewhere.

Instead of setting your reminder or alarm to leave or stop what you're doing immediately, set two reminders, one to let you know it's time to wind down or get ready and another to let you know it's time to go or begin your next task.

In addition, it's a good idea to give yourself a break between tasks where you get up, stretch, grab something to eat, or just walk around a little bit. What is important during these breaks is not to start anything new or begin social media scrolling on your phone.

Create Realistic Estimations of Time

One of the biggest challenges people with ADHD face is not that they're lazy; it's that they take on too much at once. An all-or-nothing mindset can cause serious panic and ultimately set you up for failure. While blocking out your time will definitely help you see what a realistic amount of work is, it's still essential to estimate the amount of time you will need to do something. This means factoring in unforeseen events, like your laptop needing an update, as well as being realistic about how long a task will take.

For people with ADHD, estimating time can be difficult, and the best way to overcome this challenge is to time yourself doing tasks. Once you have completed them several times, you'll be able to ascertain an average and add your time buffer to this average timeframe.

Change Your Perspective and Expectations

It's important to change your perspective about time and your expectations of how much you can do with your time. Whether you're in the midst of a time crisis or simply don't know how to manage your time effectively, changing your perspective will allow you to take a deep breath and reframe the situation.

Changing your perspective can be done by:

- Slowing things down and allowing yourself to stop panicking or feeling anxious about time.

- Delegating tasks that are not essential for you to do.

- Recalling a time when you could gain control of your time.

- Working things backward rather than forward, from your goal to your milestones, so that you can allocate enough time to tasks.

- Rewarding yourself for tasks that are completed.

- Setting time limits for social media.

Finally, I'd like you to know that even neurotypical people have issues with time. In fact, men, in general, find time management and tasks that require multiple steps or task-switching challenging.

This is because boys are not taught these skills when they are younger because of societal gender roles and stereotypes. Not being taught these skills instills certain behaviors in boys that are often carried through into adulthood. The good news is that behaviors can be changed, and you have the power to reclaim your time management skills.

A Word on Being Organized

Being organized with your time and space is the key to becoming efficiently productive. Remember, being organized doesn't mean having a meticulously clean space; it simply means finding a system that works for you.

When you create an organized environment, you spend less time looking for things and more time completing the tasks required to be productive and achieve your goals.

This is what an organization can look like:

- keeping track of your progress

- using calendars and mind maps efficiently

- creating to-do lists and keeping them up-to-date

- being accountable for your actions and changing negative behaviors

- actively eliminating distractions

- using timers and reminders

- maintaining a clean environment

- using labels to find things easily

- placing tasks, like emails, in digital folders and clearing out things that have already been done

- taking sufficient breaks between tasks

- setting SMART goals

Goal Setting for Men With ADHD

ADHD is something you're going to have for your entire life. For you to truly unlock your ADHD superpowers, you're going to need to work toward your strengths, setting goals that will help you develop and grow throughout your entire adult life.

As mentioned in Chapter 4, setting SMART goals is still the most effective way to achieve what you want to achieve in life. However, it's critical that you back these goals up with action, and this is where the ADHD brain can sometimes derail your plans.

There are six superpower skills you can use to empower yourself to take action and achieve your goals:

Skill 1: Focus on Your Strengths

It's important that you focus on your strengths and not your weaknesses. This doesn't mean you can't work on your weaknesses; it simply means you shouldn't focus on the things you believe you can't do.

Negative belief systems can cause issues for you, adversely affect your behaviors, and make you feel terrible about yourself. Focusing on the positive, however, will ensure you're celebrating all of the things you can do.

Skill 2: Make Your Goals Your Own

If you're working toward someone else's goals, you're not going to see the value in them when they're achieved. You need to take the time to define what success means to you so that you can set goals that have a purpose for *your* life. These goals can be broken down into different life areas, including your hobbies, health, fitness, career, etc.

Skill 3: Have Milestones

Part of setting SMART goals is creating milestones, but even these can overwhelm the ADHD brain. Make sure that when you set goals, you are time-blocking your milestones, organizing them into a group of manageable tasks per time slot.

You can ask yourself the following questions when setting milestones:

- What is the shortest amount of time I need to achieve this milestone?

- How many milestones are needed to achieve my goal?

- What can I do when I feel overwhelmed or procrastinate?

- If I do this task now, how much closer am I to my goal?

Skill 4: Learn Self-Discipline, Not Motivation

Motivation is a temporary emotion, which is why so many people start a goal and never achieve it. When setting goals, you're also going to need to determine how you're going to build self-discipline so that you continue achieving milestones and reach your ultimate goal.

Without self-discipline, you'll find it really difficult to overcome obstacles. Motivation simply isn't going to cut it because feeling motivated relies on dopamine, and as you know, most ADHD brains are dopamine-deficient.

Skill 5: Manage Your Mood Effectively

Changing your perspectives and learning to manage your outlook on life will positively affect your behaviors. As such, it's critical that you actively control your mood, choosing to regulate your emotions and see the positive in every situation you're facing.

Be careful with your words because what you say can also affect how well you're able to focus. The old adage by Henry Ford, "Whether you think you can, or you think you can't, you're right," is extremely pertinent to people with ADHD.

Skill 6: Build Healthy Habits

Your lifestyle will have a profound effect on your ability to achieve your goals and function in life. Ensuring that you are getting enough sleep, eating a varied and healthy diet, getting exercise, and spending time in nature are all necessary to help you manage stress and have a healthy body and mind.

Evaluating your processes and behaviors, instituting time management strategies, and ensuring you are effectively managing your stress will help you deal with the symptoms of ADHD and ensure you set yourself up for success.

Chapter 6

Boosting Your Emotional Quotient (EQ)

There is no separation of mind and emotions; emotions, thinking, and learning are all linked.

– Eric Jensen

A lot of focus is placed on intellectual quotient (IQ) when kids are growing up. While some parents encourage emotional regulation, empathy, and emotional awareness, often these skills are overlooked.

For men with ADHD, emotional regulation can be one of the most disregarded facets of having the condition. Emotional outbursts and an inability to empathize fully with others are often labeled as symptoms of ADHD. When little boys grow into men, however, deficits in EQ can cause many problems, not just in personal relationships but in the workplace too.

Before getting into the reasons why EQ is important and the strategies available to help you develop your EQ, you need to understand the difference between IQ and EQ.

IQ Versus EQ

IQ (intellectual quotient) is a measurable and standardized score for ascertaining a person's intelligence achieved via a test. An IQ test aims to accurately assess a person's cognitive capacity for reasoning and thinking. While it has been seen as controversial over the years, it is still a measure of intelligence for people across age groups.

EQ (emotional quotient), on the other hand, is a measure of how capable a person is of identifying their own emotions as well as those of others. Higher levels of EQ help people distinguish between their emotions, feelings, and moods and are used as a guide for social behaviors when interacting with other people.

The differences between EQ and IQ are as follows:

- The testing processes are both standardized, but each test requires participants to solve different questions about emotions and intelligence.

- EQ directly relates to a person's ability to succeed in life, whereas IQ relates to a person's ability to succeed academically.

- People are born with an IQ, whereas EQ is learned and acquired throughout life.

- People with an adequate EQ have great social relationships as they can express their emotions and perceive others'. A high IQ allows for a deeper understanding of data and information as well as its processing.

Emotional dysregulation occurs in people with ADHD because of executive dysfunction issues, stress, medication side effects, learned behaviors, and impulsiveness. When a person experiences emotional dysregulation, they have a hard time identifying and managing their own emotions and feelings, as well as ascertaining what other people are feeling.

Emotional outbursts, a perceived lack of empathy, and anxiety all affect a person's ability to form healthy, functioning social and personal relationships. This social exclusion and isolation can become problematic as a person often becomes depressed, which compounds their dysregulation as they don't have a chance to practice their EQ skills.

Why Emotional Regulation Is Needed for Well-Being

How we act when feeling our emotions is often the inner compass that guides us in our social interactions and building relationships. Not processing our emotions properly can cause all sorts of issues for us, not just because of our reactions but also because of how others perceive us as a result of them.

Added to this, we may act or interact incorrectly when trying to judge how others are feeling, or we simply cannot put ourselves in another person's position to empathize with them.

Emotional regulation occurs in three stages:

1. The initiating of emotions—an emotional trigger.

2. The inhibition of actions—acting, not reacting, to emotions.

3. The modulation of responses—understanding why there was an emotion.

With ADHD, steps two and three are often interrupted, and as such, an emotion is initiated with a resultant reaction occurring. In other words, we break the regulation chain, creating dysregulated emotions.

The reasons for this are not clear. They could relate to the way the ADHD brain processes stimuli or might be learned behavior. What is important to know is that emotional dysregulation occurs more often in ADHD men.

Emotional regulation acts as a modifier or buffer that helps us filter out what is essential to our safety and mental well-being and what is not. When we are dysregulated, we cannot discern what is safe, and as such, we live in a perpetual state of anxiety. When we become emotionally intelligent, we learn to regulate our emotions, lowering our anxiety and boosting our social relationships and feelings of belonging.

Other benefits of emotional regulation include:

- improved physical and mental well-being

- better performance at work

- better interpersonal and intrapersonal relationships

- greater self-awareness

Once you know the benefits of emotional regulation and can understand why being emotionally dysregulated affects your EQ, it becomes easy to assign a purpose to the strategies you will use to improve your emotional intelligence.

Strategies for Improving Emotional Intelligence

Before we dive into the strategies you can use to improve your emotional intelligence, let's take a look at the four attributes associated with EQ:

1. **The ability to self-manage:** When you are in control of your impulses, you're better able to manage your behaviors. Self-management is developed by finding healthy ways to control your emotions, take the initiative and responsibility for your actions, and follow through with what you have promised.

2. **The ability to be self-aware:** Being self-aware is the art of recognizing your emotions and how they may affect your behavior, thoughts, and interactions.

3. **The ability to be socially aware:** Empathy is the primary sign of social awareness, but other signs include being able to notice social cues, read the room, and be socially comfortable.

4. **The ability to manage relationships:** Finally, EQ is being able to maintain great relationships through proper conflict resolution, communication, and the ability to inspire others.

These attributes are directly linked to the four critical skills you require to develop to improve your EQ. These strategies are purely informational for now, but there are exercises in Chapter 7 that will assist in building upon your EQ.

Self-Management

To improve your EQ, you first need to be able to identify your emotions. Once you know what your emotions are, you can then make good decisions about what to do with them and how to resolve them constructively.

Often, stress overwhelms those of us with ADHD, and it can be very difficult to make a rational decision when we are stressed and emotional. You should acknowledge that while emotions are needed to keep us safe, a lot of the time, they're not rational or even factual.

Because of the stress we're carrying around with us, reacting to something based on perception can be very detrimental to personal relationships. Others may begin to view us as irrational or unpredictable.

Most of the time, our emotions have more to do with ourselves than other people. By learning to self-manage, we have the unique opportunity to work on our thoughts and behaviors rather than externalizing them and lashing out at others. Managing stress, therefore, is the primary focus and strategy required when learning self-management as a skill for EQ development.

Self-Awareness

Managing stress is a great way to begin self-managing. However, you will also need to be aware of your emotional experiences, your perception of life, what is triggering your emotions, and consistently be introspective so that you can deal with your thought patterns.

All of these qualities can be learned and are part of self-awareness. You must acknowledge that your emotions are not horrible experiences that happen to you. They are, in fact, valuable assets you can use in your life to develop yourself as well as your relationships.

Distancing yourself from your emotions is counterproductive, as is not taking responsibility for your actions when you don't manage your responses. However, if you aren't self-aware, understanding your emotions in a way that helps you respond appropriately can be difficult.

Social Awareness

Being socially aware is a key component to developing empathy, which is a fundamental aspect of EQ. You will need to learn to read cues in social settings so that you can assess the emotional state of others.

But social awareness goes beyond verbal communication; becoming aware of nonverbal cues is equally important. This requires concentration and a willingness to "read the room" before interrupting or sharing your point of view.

Relationship Management

The final piece to developing your EQ is to learn relationship management. Your relationships go beyond romantic ones and extend to your close friends and family too. People with ADHD can often have great social relationships and be the life of the party, but their close relationships suffer.

This is because we aren't comfortable showing acquaintances our true selves, but we are comfortable with our loved ones seeing the worst parts of us.

Part of relationship management is regulating our emotions so that we can communicate how we are feeling, but it is also the ability to see things from another person's perspective.

This is why relationship management is the final piece of the EQ puzzle. We have to self-manage, be self-aware, and develop empathy to have healthy close relationships.

Managing Stress

As you know, many men with ADHD live in a state of constant stress. Difficulty remaining focused, being surrounded by too many stimuli to process, being mindful of behaviors and moods, and the inability to remain still can all contribute to this stress and increase anxiety.

In addition, the desire to live up to others' expectations of us and feeling guilty when we don't succeed can just compound our stress. Managing our stress is a crucial facet of our life that will help us not only achieve our goals but also effectively regulate our emotions. However, for people with ADHD, normal techniques like meditation may not be enough.

Your first line of defense against stress should be to use tried-and-tested methods like:

- closing your eyes and focusing on your breath for a count of 20

- stretching for five minutes

- walking around for five minutes

If these techniques don't work, try the steps below on a daily basis to help effectively manage the stress caused by ADHD.

1. Don't Live In Denial

Blaming your behaviors on ADHD is not going to help you in the long run. You have to acknowledge your ADHD, get a proper diagnosis, keep up-to-date with your treatment plan, and work toward your goals.

2. Know Your Options

ADHD is no longer a one-treatment condition, and you have a world of treatment options available to you. For some people, medication is an absolute necessity, but for others, therapy, proper planning, and time management are enough to help you live a happy, functioning life.

3. Acknowledge that Time Isn't Fluid

Time may be fluid for you, but for other people, it is not. If you're working for someone who is flexible, you can negotiate and come to a compromise. If you're working for someone who is very rigid about timescales, explain that you sometimes have difficulty with them due to your ADHD. You could say you will implement your own reminder system but would appreciate their support (or another colleague's help) to keep you on track.

4. Set Clear Boundaries

There is absolutely no shame in having ADHD. Often, the best way to reduce your stress is to set boundaries and ask others to respect them. If you're easily distracted and working on developing your focus, speak to the people around you. Ask them to make sure they do not contribute to your distractions or request that others ensure you adhere to your reminders and alarms.

5. Embrace Structure and Routine

Structure and routine will be two of the most useful tools you develop as a man with ADHD. Make sure that you are reframing your point of view on structure and routine, moving away from the belief that they create a boring or mundane life. Routine is great—it stabilizes your body's rhythms, increases sleep quality, and reduces anxiety.

6. Set Aside Time for Fun

No one is saying you can't have fun and should just move from one routine or task to the next. It's important that you take time to do the things you love doing so that you can unwind and prevent yourself from burning out.

7. Remain Aware

It's easy to become comfortable or complacent when new routines are created and they work. Yet the nature of ADHD and the fact that most people have developed poor habits throughout their lives make it easy to slip back into old ways.

Learning to self-regulate and become emotionally intelligent are invaluable skills for anyone, but they are especially essential for men with ADHD. Our upbringing, societal constructs of how little boys are meant to act, and a brain that doesn't function neurotypically all contribute to lowered EQ. The brain, however, can change, and with training and awareness, EQ can be improved so that every ADHD man can reap the benefits of emotional intelligence.

Part 3

Improved Memory and Functioning

Chapter 7

The Power of Neuroplasticity

If we wanted to change the situation, we first had to change ourselves. And to change ourselves effectively, we first had to change our perceptions.
– Stephen Covey

Our brain's ability to adapt, change, and develop is called neuroplasticity. In the past, it was thought that neuroplasticity stopped by the time we reached adolescence and that the brain had no more capacity to learn new skills.

It was later discovered that the brain's ability to adapt, change, reorganize information, and even grow new neural networks is a lifelong capability. This is good news for people with ADHD because it means you can choose to develop new skills to help you manage the symptoms of your condition.

Neuroplasticity is categorized into two parts:

1. **Functional plasticity:** The ability of the brain to move functions from damaged or underdeveloped areas to functioning areas.

2. **Structural plasticity:** The ability to change the physical structure of the brain as a result of learning new things.

The benefits of neuroplasticity include:

- learning new things and retaining this information

- improving and enhancing cognitive functions

- recovering from brain injuries

- strengthening areas that are not functioning correctly

- improving brain fitness

Once you know that neuroplasticity is beneficial to you and has the potential to improve the quality of your life, you can begin to set goals for yourself and your self-development.

A Word on Self-Love and Self-Growth

Men with ADHD can sometimes be hypercritical of themselves. We fight our bodies and our brains. This isn't fair because our brains work differently than neurotypical ones, and we have our own superpowers we could be tapping into. Yet we're too busy hating ourselves and listening to the inner critic in our minds.

All of this means that there are many of us walking around preconditioned to believe that self-growth and self-development are things that need to be done without self-love. We only believe that we are meant to be proud of ourselves when we get things right or when we're striving for the closest definition of perfection we can reach.

Human beings are not designed to be perfect. In fact, it is in our very design to be imperfect because it is only through our mistakes that we ever learn, develop, and grow. Before you do the exercises below to learn to manage your symptoms and develop your mind, I want you to know that you *should* love yourself exactly where you are.

It's perfectly acceptable to celebrate your successes and also to honor how far you've traveled and how much adversity you've overcome. Being loved and loving yourself is a powerful motivator. Plus, when you love yourself, you're far more likely to want to become the best person you can be.

The exercises below are based on cognitive behavioral therapy (CBT) and dialectical behavior therapy (DBT) techniques, which are incredibly effective in the management of the symptoms of ADHD.

Exercise 1: Improve Working Memory

This exercise is designed to train your brain in word retrieval as well as develop critical thinking and neural agility. Fill in the form below and practice this exercise daily. Remember to add new words in the blank columns below so that your brain is challenged every time you do the exercise.

The Power of Neuroplasticity

Question	Answer	Spell Both Words Backward
What rhymes with cat?		
What rhymes with jar?		
What rhymes with hair?		
What rhymes with gate?		
What rhymes with mouse?		
What is the opposite of fast?		
What is the opposite of short?		
What is the opposite of hot?		
What is the opposite of up?		

Question	Answer	Spell the Answer Backward
Name a color		
Name a sport		
Name a vegetable		
Name a wild animal		
What is the 7th month of the year?		
What is the 4th month of the year?		
What is the 10th month of the year?		
What is your name?		
What is the name of one of your pets?		

Exercise 2: ADHD Brain Training

This activity is designed not only to train your brain, but also to assist you in learning how to control your frustration and push through obstacles and challenging situations. Trust me when I say this exercise can be extremely frustrating!

Completing this exercise will help your mind begin to focus on smaller details, honing in on what you're asking it to focus on rather than the bigger picture. Try to persevere, and over time, your brain will begin to find new ways to complete the tasks assigned to it.

Instructions

- Get two pieces of blank paper.

- Place one sheet of paper on your right and the other on your left.

- Get two pencils, placing one in each hand.

- Now, simultaneously draw a vertical line on each piece of paper using both your left and right hands.

- Repeat this three times.

- Next, draw a triangle with both hands. If this is too easy for you, draw a triangle with one hand and a square with the other.

- Now, draw a circle with both hands. If this is too easy for you, draw a circle with one hand and a triangle with the other.

- Next, draw a square with both hands. If this is too easy for you, draw a circle with your other hand.

- Are you still with me? Things are about to get a little more challenging...

- Draw a circle on one page, a square on the other page, and lift your foot off the floor at the same time.

- Now switch the pattern assigned to each hand and your foot.

If you find yourself becoming overly frustrated, slow it down, find the humor in the exercise, and remind yourself that even neurotypicals find this exercise to be extremely challenging.

Exercise 3: Improving Focus and Concentration

This exercise is designed to help you focus and concentrate, even with visual stimulation present. Try to complete one line every day of the week, and then use Google to find similar worksheets.

The first column is the letter or number you need to find. Subsequent columns will contain visually similar numbers or letters that you will need to filter out.

A	d	d	d	d	d	a	d	d	d	d	d	d	d	d	d	a	d	a	d	d	d	d	d	d
d	b	b	b	b	b	b	b	b	b	b	b	d	b	b	b	b	b	b	b	b	b	d	b	b	b
6	9	9	9	9	9	9	9	9	9	9	9	6	9	9	9	9	9	9	9	9	9	6	9	9
9	6	6	6	6	6	6	6	9	6	6	6	6	6	6	6	6	6	9	6	9	6	6	6
p	q	q	q	q	q	q	p	q	q	q	q	q	q	q	q	q	q	q	p	q	q	q	q
3	8	8	8	8	8	8	8	8	8	8	8	8	3	8	8	8	8	8	8	8	8	3	8
l	i	i	i	i	i	i	i	i	i	l	i	i	i	l	i	l	i	i	i	i	i	i

Exercise 4: Building Empathy

This worksheet is designed to help you see things from another person's perspective. Once you can begin to empathize with others, it is easier to look at your own behaviors and words and how they are affecting other people.

When someone has confronted you about your behavior, completing this worksheet before you react is an amazing way to build emotional intelligence and a great relationship.

A note on this exercise: Please remember that becoming empathetic does not mean agreeing with everyone or accepting behaviors that are toxic for you. It simply means understanding that people see the world differently from you and then deciding what the appropriate response is for you.

Instructions

- Get your journal or a piece of paper and a pen or pencil.

- Try to calm your mind and ground yourself in the present by focusing on your breath.

- When you are ready, recall a situation that caused conflict or in which you were unable to understand a person's reaction to your behavior.

- Write this situation down at the top of your page.

- Now, take a moment to think about what you were thinking just before you acted.

- Write your thoughts down.

- Next, take a moment to think about how you felt at that moment.

- Write this down.

- Think about how you acted or reacted at that moment.

- Write this down.

- Finally, think about the consequences of your actions at that moment.

- If you begin to feel irritated, frustrated, or emotional at any point, stop and return your focus to your breath.

- Once you are calm, repeat the steps above, but replace your thoughts, feelings, and actions with those of the other person.

Here is an example:

I interrupted a friend while they were talking about something important to them. I thought they had been talking for a while. I felt that the conversation was boring and wanted to speak about something more interesting to me. I acted by stepping into the conversation and speaking over my friend. The consequence of my actions was that my friend got upset and walked away from the conversation.

Reverse this so that you can see it from the other person's perspective.

My friend interrupted me while I was talking about something important to me. I thought it was disrespectful. I felt disrespected at that moment and became angry and hurt. I stepped away from the conversation because I didn't want to lash out, hurt my friend's feelings, or embarrass anyone.

In reversing the situation, it is apparent that the behavior caused the other person emotional pain. Even if you don't understand why it caused them pain, you can understand their reaction better because you know what emotional pain feels like.

Exercise 5: Managing Anxiety—RAIN

Mindfulness is the state of being able to observe our thoughts without judgment or rationality, creating a sense of awareness about how we feel without an emotional response occurring.

As you know from reading the previous chapters, being mindful is really important when dealing with and managing anxiety effectively. RAIN is a mindfulness practice that helps your mind stay grounded in the present, especially when you're experiencing thoughts and emotions that may be uncomfortable.

It stands for recognize, allow, investigate, and nurture.

Using the table below, fill in your anxious thought spiral in the RAIN section in exercise 8 and follow the instructions.

Recognize	Seek to uncover the thought you're having that is causing you anxiety. Recognize this thought consciously, as well as the feelings you're having. Name your feelings out loud or say them silently to yourself.
Allow	Observe yourself as if you were outside of your body. Imagine yourself as an actor, and you're watching yourself play out a scene. Let go of your judgments and allow yourself to feel whatever it is you're feeling.
Investigate	Notice your thoughts in detail. What words are being used? Where do you believe your thoughts and feelings are coming from? Take a moment to reflect on what you need in this moment.
Nurture	Begin to comfort yourself, expressing words of acceptance, self-love, and gratitude. Let yourself know that you're okay, that you are loved, and that emotions only last 90 seconds. Take deep breaths, letting healing, cleansing air into your body, and exhaling your anxiety.

Exercise 6: Self-Regulation Exercise—Mindfulness Meditation

Because the ADHD brain is often overstimulated, it can become easy to feel overwhelmed by the emotional responses to external and internal stimuli. Mindfulness meditation, as you know, is a fantastic way to quiet and calm the ADHD mind before reacting to our emotions and is a cornerstone of self-regulation.

In the beginning stages of learning how to practice mindfulness meditation, you may want to allocate a specifically dedicated space that you keep clean and free of clutter. If you live with other people, you should ask them not to disturb you during your meditation time.

1. Sit in a comfortable, quiet space. Straighten your back and face forward. Make sure that you're not too relaxed in your seating posture; you don't want to fall asleep!

    If sitting on the floor is not for you, you can sit in a comfortable, upright chair that supports your back. Make sure your feet can touch the ground, and place the soles of your feet flat on the floor.

    Place the palms of your hands flat on your thighs and close your eyes if you would like to.

    Now, take a deep breath in through your nose. Inhale for a count of four, and exhale through your mouth for a count of four.

    Repeat these circular cleansing breaths five times.

2. As I mentioned before, you do not have to clear your mind. In fact, it's very normal for your thoughts to wander, especially when you're trying not to think of anything.

Instead of frustrating yourself trying to clear your mind, observe your thoughts and allow them to pass naturally.

If you find yourself fixating or ruminating on one thought, acknowledge it without judgment and then return your attention to your breath.

Consciously take a moment to inhale for a count of four through your nose and exhale for a count of four through your mouth, repeating this process five times.

If the thought persists, choose to replace it with a mantra or saying.

Keep it simple, instructing your body to "breathe in and breathe out," or simply ask yourself to be calm while focusing on your breath.

3. Finally, be kind to yourself.

The reality is that you have ADHD and have spent your whole life giving in to your urges or trying to release your energy by fidgeting and moving.

If you find that the urge to scratch, fidget, or twitch is overwhelming, allow yourself to do it and then return to your practice.

Over time, these urges will diminish, and you will begin to notice that the time between them begins to lengthen.

When starting your mindfulness meditation practices, try to aim for five minutes of remaining seated and focusing on your breath. Once you have built a tolerance for these five minutes, add another session to your day, instead of extending your time in meditation. Your goal should be to have three five-minute mindfulness meditation slots during your day.

Exercise 7: Time Management Exercise—Time Blocking

The worksheet below is designed to help you effectively time-block your day so you are not overwhelmed by your tasks. This can be used in conjunction with a calendar that will remind you to shift slots or blocks.

Feel free to label blocks 1 through 4, anything you like. For example, block 1 could be the morning routine; block 2 could be prioritized work tasks; block 3 could be non-priority work tasks and home-priority tasks, and so on.

The blocks that should *not* be changed are the goal for the day and the sleep routine blocks.

Day: Monday	
My goal today is: Arrive at work on time	
Block 1	7:00 – Wake up and walk the dog
	7:30 – Have breakfast and make lunch
	8:00 – Drive to work
	9:00 – Arrive at office and attend morning briefing
	9:30 – Check and respond to emails
	BREAK
Block 2	11:00 – Finance meeting
	12:00 –Lunch
	13:00-15:30 – Regional meeting
	BREAK
Block 3	16:00 – Go to the grocery store
	16:30 - Drive home
	17:30 – Prepare and have dinner
	BREAK
Block 4	19:00 – Family time
	20:00 – Go for a walk
	21:00 – Read a book
Sleep Routine	22:00 – 23:00 • Hygiene ritual • Meditation • Stretching exercises • Set the sleep environment

Jimmy Taylor

Day:	
My goal today is:	
Block 1	
	BREAK
Block 2	
	BREAK
Block 3	
	BREAK
Block 4	
Sleep Routine	Start time: • • • •

Exercise 8: Calm the Overthinking Brain by Decluttering

Brain decluttering can also be called brain dumping, and it is an effective way to clear your mind of all of the thoughts you have surrounding your pending tasks for the day ahead.

Here is an example of what a completed brain dump looks like. A blank version, plus more instructions, are below this table so you can copy it and do this process regularly.

Work through one category at a time.

Brain Dump Worksheet

Category 1: Home	Category 2: Work
- Do the laundry more often	- Prioritize my workload
- Set up direct debits for paying bills	- Arrive on time every day
- I feel overwhelmed by everything after working all day	- Confide in someone about my ADHD –hopefully, it will help
- Get the kids to do some chores	- I feel like I look disorganized most of the time
Category 3: Family/Kids	**Category 4: Me**
- Spend more quality time with the kids	- I need to find other ways to relax and switch off my mind
- Lose my patience less with my partner	- Get back into hobbies I had when I was younger
- Worried things are getting too much and it will affect my family	- Connect more with old friends
- Visit my parents more	- Talk more about what's going on with me

Brain Dump Worksheet

Using the table provided below, write down all of your thoughts and pending tasks pertaining to the areas of your life.

Complete one category at a time.

Category 1: Home	Category 2: Work
Category 3: Family/Kids	Category 4: Me

Your brain dump information will then be used to complete the following exercise.

Exercise 9: Priority List

Once you have written down all of your thoughts and tasks for one specific category, highlight or circle any important tasks and move them to the first block in the priority list below. Any remaining tasks should go in the "Non-priority tasks" section. Now write the priority tasks that you want to focus on in the "Activities to be added to the time blocking sheet." Any negative or critical thoughts should be written in the final block, so that you can use the RAIN exercise to investigate and deal with the feelings and thoughts you're having.

Other thoughts can be discarded or ignored. A great way to deal with all of the clutter in your mind once you have written it out on this worksheet is to tear up the exercise page and take five minutes for mindfulness meditation.

Priority List

Priority tasks	1
	2
	3
	4
	5
	6

Non-Priority tasks	1
	2
	3
	4
	5
	6
Activities to be added to the time blocking sheet:	1
	2
	3
	4
	5
	6
Write down any negative or critical thoughts here to use the RAIN exercise with.	1
	2
	3
	4
	5
	6

As previously mentioned, these exercises are based on (CBT) and (DBT) which are proven techniques to manage ADHD symptoms. Take the time to incorporate one exercise at a time in your daily routine. You may want to start with the easiest one. When you master it, you can move to the next exercise, and so on. Once you get into the habit of doing these exercises daily, it will help you manage your ADHD positively so that you can begin to thrive.

Chapter 8

Thriving With ADHD

Lineage, personality, and environment may shape you, but they do not define your full potential.
– Mollie Marti

ADHD is a lifelong condition with no cure. This doesn't mean you need to suffer with your symptoms, though. With therapy, self-care, medication, and a willingness to work on your behaviors, you can begin to thrive with ADHD.

Remember, ADHD comes with its own set of superpowers, but it's up to you to unlock them by using the resources available to you. This last chapter is dedicated to the self-care and lifestyle changes you can make to help enhance your superpowers to become the best man you can possibly be.

Before you read the information below, I'd like you to take a moment to remind yourself that your definition of success is yours alone. You don't need to be anyone else, nor do you have to build a life that isn't uniquely yours.

Why Self-Care Is Important

Self-care is extremely important for men with ADHD to help reduce the symptoms of the condition and bring focus to taking care of our bodies and minds. Concentrating on our symptoms and having to deal with an enormous amount of stimuli daily can be mentally and physically exhausting. When we neglect our bodies, it can become even harder to focus on everyday tasks. Prioritizing self-care is a form of self-love that will greatly improve our quality of life and is one of the critical steps in achieving success when it comes to our goals for ourselves.

Many men think that self-care is something only women do, and when asked, they usually define it as trips to the spa, massages, pedicures, and so on. Now, there is absolutely nothing wrong with men participating in these activities. In fact, I encourage you to try at least one of these every month. But they are an added bonus on top of a great self-care routine.

Self-care includes:

- creating a great sleep routine for good sleep

- getting enough exercise

- eating nutritious, healthy meals

- reducing clutter in your home and mind

- creating a daily schedule that is routine

- practicing exercises for improved concentration, emotional regulation, and organization

In addition to the list above, self-care is the prioritization of your needs so that you can build self-love and self-esteem.

Healthy Lifestyle Habits for Men With ADHD

Now that you know why self-care is important, let's break down each area so it's easier for you to incorporate them into your life.

Sleep and Sleep Routines

Getting enough quality sleep is essential for the health of your brain and body. For people with ADHD, sleep is often viewed as a waste of time, but proper, restorative sleep helps with mood regulation, attention span, and memory, as well as the healing of the body.

Creating a sleep routine that facilitates proper restorative sleep can be challenging for men with ADHD, as poor habits may have led to circadian rhythm issues. The great news is that with a little persistence, you can reclaim your sleep and reap the benefits of proper rest.

Here are a few tips:

1. Move away from technology and screens an hour before your bedtime. If you haven't set a time to get into bed, do it now.

2. Make sure you're free of distractions an hour before you go to sleep. These distractions can include scrolling through social media, gaming, or starting the next episode of your favorite show. Instead, choose to do the quick chores that need to be done in your home, like packing the dishwasher or doing a brief tidy-up. That way, you can wake up to a clean, orderly home the next day, ensuring you can stay on track with your schedule.

Set a timer for 30 minutes for these tasks and assign them to the first half of your sleep routine.

3. The last 30 minutes of your sleep routine should include personal hygiene, including a warm bath or shower, brushing your teeth, reading, and meditating.

4. Set a reminder to get into bed and stick to it. Even if you lie in the dark for a while, that's fine. The point is to allow your mind and body to begin training themselves to go to sleep earlier.

If you've been practicing great sleep hygiene for more than a month and your mind is still resisting sleep, you may want to consider a melatonin supplement. Always consult with your healthcare professional before taking new medications. Make sure you read the instructions for your melatonin, take it a few hours before you sleep, and understand that long-term melatonin use can hinder sleep routines.

Exercise for Men With ADHD

Getting sufficient exercise is beneficial for everyone, but for the ADHD man, it allows for the release of pent-up energy and provides an external outlet for internalized hyperactivity symptoms.

For men with ADHD, it's important to find interesting, engaging, and exciting exercise options that will keep them from getting bored. When coupled with great nutrition, exercise is one of the most powerful tools for helping to release energy, regulate mood, and deal with stress and anxiety.

1. Set realistic exercise goals for yourself, especially if you are currently sedentary. Aim for 15 minutes of vigorous exercise every second day to begin with, working your way up to a maximum of one hour every day of the week. Change your routines and incorporate different types of exercise so that you remain interested.

2. Make sure your exercise is moderate to vigorous. You should be breathing hard but not exhausted.

3. Do activities that involve different muscle groups and build upon motor skills at least twice a week. These can include martial arts, dancing, or ball sports.

Make sure to nourish your body properly both before and after working out, and look for natural forms of protein and amino acids rather than consuming convenient shakes or protein bars. These convenience products often contain ingredients that exacerbate hyperactive symptoms.

Nutrition for Men With ADHD

The ADHD brain requires certain vitamins and minerals in higher quantities. As the brain is made up mostly of fat, which is responsible for neural brain signaling, an increase in omega-3 fatty acids is essential for the ADHD brain.

Nutrients like zinc, iron, and vitamin D are also essential for proper brain signaling, and these nutrients are often lacking in modern convenience foods. One of the biggest challenges men with ADHD face is the inability to complete multi-step tasks, making cooking a real chore. It is, however, essential to learn how to cook properly so that you can nourish your body. Once you find the excitement and creativity in cooking, it can be a lot of fun.

1. Start small when making dietary changes. Getting rid of everything unhealthy all at once can feel overwhelming or like a punishment.

2. Significantly reduce stimulant foods like coffee, tea, and energy drinks. Eliminating these is actually best, but a reduction can also make a difference.

3. Make sure you're getting enough zinc, iron, and vitamin D from natural sources like fatty fish, avocados, leafy greens, and eggs.

4. Become mindful of and eliminate foods that trigger symptoms or make them worse.

Everyone's body is different regarding nutrition, but general eating guidelines are to make sure you're consuming larger meals in the middle of the day, fueling your body properly before and after exercise, and eating mineral- and nutrition-rich foods.

Healthy Support Systems

Building a healthy support system is important as it can help you through tough times, be there when you want to bounce ideas off someone, provide positive feedback, and celebrate your victories.

Structured support systems are often in the form of support groups that are geared toward helping people with ADHD and may include professionals who offer guidance and resources. Informal support systems usually include friends and family who understand or empathize with your struggles and provide emotional and physical aid.

Having both of these support systems in your life will help you get the most out of building a positive group of people. They will assist you in reaching your goals and in dealing with the specific challenges you face.

With these people around you, you can gain valuable insights and empower yourself in how to manage your symptoms properly. All of this, of course, means being able to thrive in your life.

The aims of joining support groups and creating a network of positively influential people in your life are:

- encouraging and maintaining new behaviors

- reinforcing good behaviors

- bringing attention to symptoms that need to be managed

- sharing knowledge and experiences

- offering emotional support

- learning empathy for other people's struggles

Success is a lonely journey if you do not have anyone to share it with. Having people in your life who can love and support you will provide you with more motivation to succeed.

Conclusion

Thriving isn't about making life comfortable, fun, and happy; it's about finding purpose and making our own unique contribution.
– Malcolm Stern

ADHD may come with a high level of stigma attached to it, and for the men who live with it, this stigma can often cause a lot of anxiety, guilt, and shame. Getting a diagnosis doesn't need to be this way, though, and finding out why life feels challenging at times is the first step in learning the tools required to unlock your ADHD superpowers.

Practicing the tools provided helps us to manage our symptoms and stick to the treatment plans. Ultimately, this will enhance our quality of life and improve everything from our ability to be productive to emotional regulation and even our relationships.

If you have just received an ADHD diagnosis, it's okay and natural to feel overwhelmed. If you've been aware of your ADHD for a while but haven't quite known where to start when it comes to at-home tools, you've taken the right steps toward your symptom management future.

Using the exercises and information available in this book, like mind mapping, time-blocking, mindfulness meditation, executive functioning, improving your EQ, etc., are great add-ons to your conventional therapy and other prescribed treatments.

Before finishing this book and putting the information and exercises into practice, I want you to know that you're not alone. There are so many men out there, some that you know of and most that you don't, who took steps to manage their ADHD. It was through this management that they found their definition of success in the same way that you can.

Olympic champion Michael Phelps was nine when he was diagnosed with severe ADHD. With his mother's guidance, Phelps used his interest in swimming to help him focus on his schoolwork, ultimately leading to successfully weaning himself off medication. Today, Phelps has 22 Olympic medals—the most any athlete has ever won.

Grammy-award singer Justin Timberlake has been public about his ADHD and OCD struggles, but also credits his success to the tools he was taught to manage his symptoms. Also, comedian and presenter Howie Mandel, with the support of his wife and parents, has overcome ADHD, becoming the spokesperson for the 'Adult ADHD is Real' campaign.

Even billionaire Bill Gates, the founder of Microsoft, has tapped into his ADHD superpowers to become one of the richest men in the world, using a lot of his wealth as a contributor to charities.

You see, living with ADHD doesn't mean you need to struggle through life. In fact, when you unlock your ADHD superpowers, learn to love yourself, and embrace your self-growth journey to gain deeper insight into just how wonderfully unique you are, ADHD has the potential to be the very source of your quest for a thriving life.

Conclusion

You now have the tools and information you need to live a life that is successful, loving, and as amazingly unique as you are. I would love to hear about your journey with ADHD and how this book has helped you, so please feel free to leave a review and a comment so that others know they're not alone.

Thank You

Thank you for purchasing my book.

I would like to ask you for a small favor. **Could you please leave a review on the platform? Leaving a review is the best way to support me as an independent author.**

Your feedback is valuable to me. It helps me write books that are aligned with your desired outcomes. I would greatly appreciate hearing from you.

Do not forget to download "Your Empowering Checklist for Success and Happiness" for free!!

If you are looking to explore self-help and personal growth, I invite you to discover my books on Amazon. They offer many tips and strategies to support your journey.

References

Alder, S. (n.d.). *Adhd Quotes*. Goodreads. https://www.goodreads.com/quotes/tag/adhd

Alhawatmeh, H. N., Rababa, M., Alfaqih, M., Albataineh, R., Hweidi, I., & Abu Awwad, A. (2022). The Benefits of Mindfulness Meditation on Trait Mindfulness, Perceived Stress, Cortisol, and C-Reactive Protein in Nursing Students: A Randomized Controlled Trial. *Advances in Medical Education and Practice, Volume 13*, 47–58. https://doi.org/10.2147/amep.s348062

Amen, D. G. (2001). *Healing ADD*. Penguin.

Asarnow, R. F., Newman, N., Weiss, R. E., & Su, E. (2021). Association of Attention-Deficit/Hyperactivity Disorder Diagnoses With Pediatric Traumatic Brain Injury. *JAMA Pediatrics*. https://doi.org/10.1001/jamapediatrics.2021.2033

Balogh, L., Pulay, A. J., & Réthelyi, J. M. (n.d.). *Genetics in the ADHD Clinic: How Can Genetic Testing Support the Current Clinical Practice?* Frontiersin. https://www.frontiersin.org/articles/10.3389/fpsyg.2022.751041/full

Beheshti, A., Chavanon, M.-L., & Christiansen, H. (2020). Emotion dysregulation in adults with attention deficit hyperactivity disorder: a meta-analysis. *BMC Psychiatry, 20*. https://doi.org/10.1186/s12888-020-2442-7

Belmont, J. (2017) *CBT Technique: Using the Triple Column Technique to Change Your Thoughts to Change Your Life!* PsychCentral. https://psychcentral.com/pro/psychoeducation/2017/07/cbt-technique-

Jimmy Taylor

using-the-triple-column-technique-to-change-your-thoughts-to-change-your-life#1

Carnegie, A. (n.d). Goodreads.
https://www.goodreads.com/quotes/122624-if-you-want-to-be-happy-set-a-goal-that

Champ, R. E., Adamou, M., & Tolchard, B. (2021). The impact of psychological theory on the treatment of Attention Deficit Hyperactivity Disorder (ADHD) in adults: A scoping review. *PLOS ONE, 16*(12), e0261247. https://doi.org/10.1371/journal.pone.0261247

Covey, S. (n.d.). *Stephen R. Covey Quotes.* Goodreads.
https://bestbookbits.com/the-7-habits-of-highly-effective-people-powerful-lessons-in-personal-change-by-stephen-covey/

Donzelli, G., Carducci, A., Llopis-Gonzalez, A., Verani, M., Llopis-Morales, A., Cioni, L., & Morales-Suárez-Varela, M. (2019). The Association between Lead and Attention-Deficit/Hyperactivity Disorder: A Systematic Review. International *Journal of Environmental Research and Public Health, 16*(3), 382. https://doi.org/10.3390/ijerph16030382

Eddings, M. (n.d.). *Adhd Quotes.* Goodreads.
https://www.goodreads.com/quotes/tag/adhd

Ford, H (n.d.). *Henry Ford Quotes.* Goodreads.
https://www.goodreads.com/author/quotes/203714.Henry_Ford

Ghaemi, S. N. (2018). After the failure of DSM: clinical research on psychiatric diagnosis. *World Psychiatry, 17*(3), 301–302.
https://doi.org/10.1002/wps.20563

Jensen, E. (n.d.). *Emotional Intelligence Quotes.* Sources of Insight.
https://sourcesofinsight.com/emotional-intelligence-quotes/

References

Attention-deficit/hyperactivity disorder (ADHD) in children - Symptoms and causes. (2019, June 25). Mayo Clinic. https://www.mayoclinic.org/diseases-conditions/adhd/symptoms-causes/syc-20350889

Mercedes, S. (n.d.). *Adhd Quotes*. Goodreads. https://www.goodreads.com/quotes/tag/adhd

Millman, D. (n.d.). *Dan Millman Quotes*. Goodreads. https://www.goodreads.com/quotes/10158365-you-don-t-have-to-control-your-thoughts-you-just-have

Marti, M. (n.d.). *Thriving Quotes*. Goodreads. https://www.goodreads.com/quotes/tag/thriving

Montagna, A., Karolis, V., Batalle, D., Counsell, S., Rutherford, M., Arulkumaran, S., Happe, F., Edwards, D., & Nosarti, C. (2020). ADHD symptoms and their neurodevelopmental correlates in children born very preterm. *PLOS ONE, 15*(3), e0224343. https://doi.org/10.1371/journal.pone.0224343

Attention-Deficit/Hyperactivity Disorder (ADHD). (2014). National Institute of Mental Health. https://www.nimh.nih.gov/health/statistics/attention-deficit-hyperactivity-disorder-adhd

Pera, G. (2022, March 12). *Sleep Deprivation: ADHD Symptoms Keeping You Awake?* Additude Magazine. https://www.additudemag.com/wired-tired-sleep-deprived/

Rai, D. (n.d.). *Dharmendra Raj Quotes*. Goodreads. https://www.goodreads.com/quotes/11137481-it-is-not-easy-to-make-things-simple---one

Roth, R. M., & Saykin, A. J. (2004). Executive dysfunction in attention-deficit/hyperactivity disorder: cognitive and neuroimaging findings.

Psychiatric Clinics of North America, 27(1), 83–96.
https://doi.org/10.1016/s0193-953x(03)00112-6

Ryu, S., Choi, Y.-J., An, H., Kwon, H.-J., Ha, M., Hong, Y.-C., Hong, S.-J., & Hwang, H.-J. (2022). Associations between Dietary Intake and Attention Deficit Hyperactivity Disorder (ADHD) Scores by Repeated Measurements in School-Age Children. *Nutrients, 14*(14), 2919. https://doi.org/10.3390/nu14142919

Sarkis, S. (2011, July 21). Do People With ADHD Cheat More? *Psychology Today.* https://www.psychologytoday.com/intl/blog/here-there-and-everywhere/201107/do-people-adhd-cheat-more

Shapiro, S. (2016, January 20). Adult ADHD and Work: Improving Executive Function: 5 strategies to improve work performance. https://www.psychologytoday.com/us/blog/the-best-strategies-for-managing-adult-adhd/201601/adult-adhd-and-work-improving-executive?amp

Silver, Dr. L. (2023, March 28). *ADHD Symptoms Or ADHD Comorbidity? Diagnosing Related Conditions.* Additude Magazine. https://www.additudemag.com/when-its-not-just-adhd/#:~:text=At%20least%20half%20of%20all

Song, P., Zha, M., Yang, Q., Zhang, Y., Li, X., & Rudan, I. (2021). The prevalence of adult attention-deficit hyperactivity disorder: A global systematic review and meta-analysis. *Journal of Global Health, 11*(04009). https://doi.org/10.7189/jogh.11.04009

Spurgeon, C. (n.d.). *Charles Spurgeon Quotes.* Brainy Quote. https://www.brainyquote.com/quotes/charles_spurgeon_132220

Stern, M. (n.d.). *Malcolm Stern Quotes.* Goodreads. https://www.goodreads.com/quotes/10335289-thriving-isn-t-about-making-life-comfortable-fun-and-happy-it-s

Stevens, T. (2006). There Is No Meaningful Relationship Between Television Exposure and Symptoms of Attention-Deficit/Hyperactivity Disorder. *PEDIATRICS, 117*(3), 665–672. https://doi.org/10.1542/peds.2005-0863

Weissenberger, S., Schonova, K., Büttiker, P., Fazio, R., Vnukova, M., Stefano, G. B., & Ptacek, R. (2021). Time Perception is a Focal Symptom of Attention-Deficit/Hyperactivity Disorder in Adults. *Medical Science Monitor, 27.* https://doi.org/10.12659/msm.933766

Wilens, T. E., & Spencer, T. J. (2010). Understanding Attention-Deficit/Hyperactivity Disorder from Childhood to Adulthood. *Postgraduate Medicine, 122*(5), 97–109. https://doi.org/10.3810/pgm.2010.09.2206

Made in the USA
Las Vegas, NV
06 February 2024

85384309R00098